***The Discovery of Talent***

*The Walter Van Dyke Bingham Lectures on the Development of Exceptional Abilities and Capacities*

# *The Discovery of Talent*

*Edited by*
*Dael Wolfle*

*The Walter Van Dyke Bingham Lectures on the Development of Exceptional Abilities and Capacities*

*Harvard University Press*
*Cambridge, Massachusetts*
*1969*

*Distributed in Great Britain by Oxford University Press, London*

*Library of Congress Catalog Card Number: 69–18046*

*Printed in the United States of America*

# *Introduction*

"Finding the talented, encouraging their advancement, making known their potentialities" serves two purposes: individuals are helped to fulfill their promise, and society is enriched. To aid individuals or to enrich society—the emphasis has sometimes been on one and sometimes on the other of these complementary goals—man has long engaged in a talent search. Many cultures, in many ages, in many parts of the world have nurtured their talented youth. Ancient China sought young scholars who could excel in the rigorous civil service examinations that selected servants of the state. The medieval Catholic Church reared many of its cardinals and at least half of its popes from among the humbly born. Indian tribes of British Columbia prepared the most skillful young hunters and fishermen for roles of leadership. These societies and others have shared the common purpose of identifying and encouraging the kinds of talent each prized most highly.

Western Europe and the United States have not only shared this common purpose but in the present century, more deliberately than men have ever done before, have also sought to understand the nature of human talent.

The eleven lectures in this volume describe both aims: to try to understand what talent is, and to try to understand how talent may be recognized and developed. The lectures do not, however, provide a fully rounded treatment of all facets of these two aims. The lecturers were not selected for that purpose, but rather to give recognition to individuals who had in some significant fashion contributed to the better identification of the talented. Each wrote of his own work or of the area in which his interest had centered. Consequently, some matters which other speakers would have chosen to emphasize are not included here, or treated only lightly. For example, it would be of interest to include a history of the means various societies have used to identify the kinds of talent each wanted to cultivate, but no one chose this topic.

Nevertheless, with different degrees of comprehensiveness and detail, the central issues were considered by one or more of the eleven lecturers. The themes they developed could be analyzed in a variety of ways. I choose to take them up under three headings:

1. The nature of human ability and the reasons for its variability.
2. The structure of human ability.
3. The methods of measuring, predicting, and fostering the development of human ability.

### *The Nature of Human Ability and the Reasons for its Variability*

Philosophers, psychologists, and educators have wrestled with the problem of defining *intelligence* or *aptitude* or *ability* or whatever other term one attaches to those qualities that permit some persons to perform socially valued tasks more accurately, more rapidly, or with greater power than do others. Some scholars have assumed the existence of an underlying aptitude which is given to a child by his genes and which exists whether or not it becomes manifest in the particular environment in which he is reared. There is justification for this position, but it often hides the importance of other variables that contribute to human accomplishment. Stalnaker was criticizing such one-sidedness when he said that "the IQ is overrated. Unfortunately, parents and even many teachers regard the IQ as an infallible and crucially significant index. As a result, they ignore the importance of the many other characteristics which contribute to attainment. In the final analysis it is not how bright one is, but what one has accomplished that counts."

Many characteristics of the life history of two men help explain why one accomplishes more than the other. Heredity, education, health, physical energy and work habits, motivation (and all that word encompasses), parental advantage, the often irrelevant aspects of physical appearance or manner of speech, and the quite unpredictable accidents that put one person in the right place at the right time—all such matters may help to explain A's success and B's failure.

Intelligence is a useful concept, but none of the lecturers attribute all of the differences in achievement to differences in intelligence. Eight of the eleven—Terman, Burt, Strong, Wolfle, Stalnaker, MacKinnon, Ghiselli, and Mackworth—explicitly point out that other factors are involved, and several of them devote most of their lectures to these other factors. Terman discusses personality traits that make for success, and Strong describes the efforts he and others have made to measure vocational interests. Burt considers the inheritance of emotional and temperamental qualities that affect the way one works and the amount one achieves. MacKinnon, Ghiselli, and Mackworth concentrate on important kinds of ability that are not well measured by any of the available tests of "intelligence."

Intelligence is not the only variable, but in a society that puts much emphasis on formal education, on the ability to deal with symbols and abstractions, and on the ability to use language effectively, it has rightly been one of the most thoroughly studied. Much of this study has centered on the long-continuing debate over the relative contributions of heredity and environment in creating differences in human achievement. Heredity and environment have each been given credit as the major contributor, and each has its supporter in these pages.

Burt is more assured than any of his colleagues on the heredity-environment problem; for him, hereditary differences far outweigh environmental differences. His analysis of the intelligence-test scores of schoolchildren leads him to conclude that "nearly 23% of the total variance appears due to nongenetic influences, i.e., to environment or to unreliability, and about 77% to genetic factors." When he makes adjustments to allow for what appear to be erroneous scores, he finds that "only about 12% (or slightly more) is apparently due to nongenetic influences and 88% to genetic factors."

Others disagree. Terman, without being statistical or quantitative about the matter, emphasizes the importance of the zeitgeist in determining the abilities that will be fostered, rewarded, developed, and hence varied. Vernon emphasizes environmental determinants, and most of the other lecturers give them substantially greater weight than does Burt.

Had other lecturers been chosen for the series, it is probable that other answers to the heredity-environment question would have been given. I recall an international conference of a dozen years ago in which a distinguished British geneticist announced that 50 percent of the variance in human ability was due to differences in heredity and 50 percent to differences in environment. I asked whether this precise balancing of importance resulted from experimental evidence or represented his best guess about a situation which admitted of no final answer. I was assured that the evidence supported the 50–50 division.

The gentleman gave the wrong answer. He was wrong for two very significant reasons, although it seems to have taken an unduly long time for us to come to understand their significance. One reason is that the relative importance of heredity or environment differs in different populations. All of the difference between two identical twins is attributable to nongenetic factors. Much of the difference between a normal child and a congenital idiot is genetically determined. The relative importance of environment increases with age. In short, the relative contributions of heredity and environment depend upon the population in which they are studied.

Most scholars would recognize this point, as does Burt, and would probably reply that they agree but that in attempting to assess the relative contributions of the two factors, they were dealing with a "normal" population, usually a population of "normal" schoolchildren. Even so, the argument has probably helped draw attention away from the wide variety of environmental variables that affect intellectual growth. In the final address of the series, Vernon offers much the most sophisticated treatment of the problem. In addition to genetic factors, he lists nine environmental determinants of children's performance on standardized tests. Expressed in terms of handicaps, they are: malnutrition and disease, perceptual deprivation in the preschool years and conceptual deprivation during school years, repression of independence and constructive play, family insecurity and lack of planfulness, female dominance, defective education, linguistic handicaps, the conceptual and grammatical structure of the child's native language, and the unattractiveness of adult roles that are visible and the resultant lowering of adolescent aspirations.

Vernon's list of environmental variables provides a good introduction to the second reason why the British geneticist was wrong in saying that exactly 50 percent of the variance could be attributed to inherited and 50 percent to environmental differences. That statement overlooked what the statisticians call interaction. The effects of heredity plus the effects of environment, each acting independently, do not account for 100 percent of the variance; the interaction between heredity and environment must also be included in the equation. As Vernon points out, it is necessary "to get away from the notion of intelligence as a definite entity, an autonomous mental faculty, which simply matures as children grow up. Rather we have to think of it in terms of a cumulative formation of more and more complex and flexible [ways of dealing with situations] which develop through interaction between the growing organism and its environment." The genetically superior infant and his less well endowed brother react differently to the sights and sounds and other stimuli that affect them both. Reacting differently, the superior infant develops a different method of responding to other environmental variables and of dealing with the information he receives. And these differential methods of reacting provide different kinds and amounts of practice in developing inherited traits or tendencies. Thus the interaction builds up. Hereditary differences influence the ways in which the child responds to the environment. Differential responses to the environment influence the manner and speed of development of inherited potentialities. By the time the child is old enough to become a subject for the psychologist's or the geneticist's investigation, a large part of what he does is no longer attributable to either variable acting alone, but must be explained in terms of their interaction.

This view of the matter—sensible and obvious as it seems now—was a long time in developing. It would not be right to say that the earlier scholars who argued as if two definite and immutable figures which add up to 100 could be found were wasting their time. But it is correct to say that the percentages are not immutable, that the problem is now formulated in a more insightful fashion, and that attention can now be turned to problems which stand a greater chance of leading to socially useful ideas for improving child development.

### *The Structure of Human Ability*

So far we have been discussing differences in human ability as if they could all be scaled along a single continuum, as if human ability were a unitary trait. That this is a gross oversimplification of the true situation has been evident for far longer than there have been systematic studies of the nature of ability. It must have been evident for millennia that the person who excelled in one kind of activity did not necessarily reach an equal standard of excellence in other kinds of activities. At least for centuries, some persons have been known as musical geniuses, others as mathematical geniuses, and still others as particularly competent in other areas. There has also been interest in those peculiar individuals who are generally considered stupid but who can remember long strings of numbers heard only once, or who perform surprisingly well in some other fashion.

Statisticians and psychologists have studied, analyzed, and interpreted these differences in an extensive literature on mental factors. Broadly speaking, there have been three schools of thought concerning the underlying structure of human ability.

One is the idea that there is a large and pervasive factor of general intelligence and a relatively restricted number of special factors. Charles Spearman did more than anyone else to establish this view.

The second theory holds that there are a number of relatively independent and more or less co-equal factors which combine in different patterns to account for the differences in performance on different kinds of tasks and tests. Among contributors to this theory, the leader was L. L. Thurstone, who was chosen to give the second lecture in the series. Unfortunately, his lecture was never delivered. Ill health forced a postponement, and Dr. Thurstone's death a few months later terminated a career of brilliant contributions to the study of human ability.

Adherents of the third position hold that intelligence consists of a large number of rather narrow or specific kinds of abilities. The name of Godfrey Thompson is most closely associated with this position.

None of the lecturers are avowed supporters of Godfrey

Thompson's theory of many highly specific factors, but both Spearman's theory of a general factor (usually symbolized by the letter *g*) and Thurstone's theory of group factors claim supporters among the eleven lecturers. Sometimes support is based on theoretical grounds, sometimes on pragmatic grounds.

Terman and Ghiselli brush the factor problem aside by saying or implying that whatever the underlying structure may be in theory, they consider the matter pragmatically and therefore treat intelligence in an unanalyzed fashion. Terman is the more specific: "Both the evidence on early mental development of historical geniuses and that obtained by follow-up of gifted subjects selected in childhood by mental tests point to the conclusion that capacity to achieve far beyond the average can be detected early in life by a well-constructed ability test that is heavily weighted with the *g* factor." Vernon, for both theoretical and practical reasons, also follows Spearman in emphasizing the *g* factor.

Among the lecturers who devote considerable attention to the underlying structure of ability, Guilford is the most positive and enthusiastic. He follows Thurstone more avidly than Thurstone ever followed his own pioneering ideas.

Guilford defines the object of his search in these words: "Each intellectual component or factor is a unique ability that is needed to do well in a certain class of tasks or tests." He identifies some 50 separate factors, which he arranges in a three-dimensional model called "the structure of intellect." On one dimension are arrayed four classes of intellectual content with which one may work: figural, symbolic, semantic, and behavioral or social. The second dimension is defined by five kinds of operation performed: evaluation, convergent thinking, divergent thinking, memorization, and cognition. "When a certain operation is applied to a certain kind of content, as many as six general kinds of products may be involved." These six products constitute the third dimension: units, classes, relations, systems, transformations, and implications. This model, with the three axes divided, respectively, into four, five, and six segments, includes 120 spaces or cells.

According to Guilford, there should be a factor for each cell. Not all have been found, but he has identified about 50. To complicate the matter, however, some of the 120 cells contain more than one factor, and so, he concludes, "we may end up with more than 120 abilities," each of which would be "a unique ability."

Vernon, whose position as the final lecturer in the series gave him an opportunity to get in the last word on several controversial points, rejected Guilford's model. He points out that the intercorrelations among tests—the prime data which the factor analysts analyze—are determined not only by the test content and whatever underlying abilities may be involved, but also "by the form or technique of the tests, its speededness, level of difficulty of the items, whether multiple-choice or creative response, whether analogies, series or classifications, and so forth," and summarizes his position by quoting Quinn McNemar's characterization of "fragmentation of ability into more and more factors of less and less importance."

There is a middle ground in this argument. It goes something like this. Factor analysis is useful in studying the interrelations among a variety of tasks or performances. The number and nature of the factors one finds depend, however, upon the nature, number, and variety of tasks or tests included in the original battery from which the intercorrelations are derived and upon the method used to factor analyze these intercorrelations. There is no unique set of factors that describes once and for all the varieties of intellectual performance. On the practical side, factor analysis helps to give an understanding of the interrelations among different kinds of performance or different tasks. But for personnel selection, or for educational or vocational guidance, little is added by going much beyond the general factor (if one believes in *g*) or a small number of group factors (if one prefers the multiple-factor approach).

In a general and qualitative fashion, one can relate this conclusion to the earlier discussion of the nature of human ability and the reasons for its variability. The determiners of human ability are multiple and the relations among them complex. They have acted in different combinations, with different effects, at different times, on different individuals. There is wide variety in the kinds of material (verbal, pictorial, arithmetical, symbolic, and so forth) that can be dealt with by human beings, and there is also wide variety in the kinds of tasks that involve these varied materials. One must therefore expect to find varying patterns of correlations when different sets of tasks, involving different types of materials, are presented to different groups of subjects. That there is no unique set of underlying factors that can "explain" all the varieties and differences in human ability is the only reasonable conclusion.

Nevertheless, there are consistencies in human performance. There are major trends or themes in human development and in education. Factor analysis provides a sometimes useful means of identifying and of coming closer to understanding these consistencies.

### *Measuring, Predicting, and Fostering the Development of Human Ability*

When Terman was young, the slogan "early ripe, early rot" was widely accepted. Egalitarianism leads to such beliefs. The precocious child is expected to burn out. The backward one is expected to be a late bloomer. The person who excels in one field is deficient in another. And of course there is some truth in these generalizations. Some bright children do not reach the levels expected of them. Others accomplish more than early indications would lead one to predict. People do have their strengths and their weaknesses.

But there is also consistency in human performance. No one has done more than Terman to demonstrate that intellectual superiority in childhood is generally followed by intellectual superiority as an adult. Who better than Terman could have started off this series of addresses with solid, empirical evidence that talented youngsters become talented adults, that the stories about the backward boyhoods of the great men of history lack foundation, that the slogan "early ripe, early rot" is in fact rot?

Terman's evidence (and, of course, the evidence from other sources) that bright children become able, productive adults, the evidence that there is consistency in human performance both over time and over a range of related tasks, makes possible not only research on the structure of ability but also makes possible, and socially useful, a variety of practical efforts to identify and cultivate talents. Several of the lecturers deal with such efforts.

Stalnaker describes "how the problem of discovering and encouraging talent on an extensive scale has actually been handled" by the National Merit Scholarship Program. Starting with about 600,000 high school juniors who took the Merit Program preliminary selection test in 1960, a succession of hurdles reduced the group a year later to about 5,000 who received college scholarships and another 30,000 who received honors or commendations. Accompanying the scholarship program is a continuing series of research studies on methods of selection and on the subsequent performance of the very superior high school students who go through the selection process. Stalnaker's data agree with Terman's in showing that the very bright tend to be superior in other respects and that their high performance continues in later years.

MacKinnon and Mackworth discuss creativity or originality. MacKinnon studied mature, professional men judged by their colleagues to be high in creativity. Architecture was the field he used to illustrate his work. In such groups, all of whose members are at least moderately intelligent, he found the relationship between intelligence, as usually measured, and rated creativity to be essentially zero. The creative architect is not necessarily more "intelligent" than the uncreative one, but somehow he uses his abilities differently. His childhood experiences and early family environment and treatment also differed typically from those of the less creative architects, as did a number of the personality traits MacKinnon investigated. But what kinds of training or experiences are effective in producing high creativity is still a puzzle. As a student, the truly creative individual may be rebellious, sometimes uncertain and in some turmoil, and thus hard for the teacher to accept. The warning to teachers is not to quell creativity by insisting on docility.

Mackworth's analysis of scientific originality differentiates between scientists who are able to solve problems and the more imaginative and seminal ones who advance scientific thought by formulating new problems. Because the latter are fewer and more precious, he goes on to discuss the arrangements, methods of support, and working relationships that might favor research productivity.

Strong and Ghiselli also depart from the general emphasis on intelligence to discuss other elements involved in career choice and performance. Strong raises questions about the role of interests, attitudes, goals, and satisfactions in determining vocational choice and in contributing to vocational success. Despite general agreement on the importance of these elements of the human makeup, Strong's lecture is evidence of how little we know about them.

Ghiselli's examinations of managerial talent show that intelligence is only one of the elements required for success, and that at the very highest levels intellectual ability may even be a detriment: "It is possible that these individuals at the very extreme high levels of capacity to deal with abstract ideas and concepts do not find in managerial activities the intellectual challenge they need." In agreement with Strong, Ghiselli also finds interests, attitudes, and personality variables significant determiners of managerial competence.

Paterson deals primarily with problems of vocational guidance and vocational training and considers both effective and successful people and some who are not. He considers the ill effects of discrimination in preventing the normal development of talent and regrets the talent that is lost to society because we fail to develop it adequately.

The urgent social problem of preventing potential talent from being killed or stunted has been coming into increasingly sharp focus in recent years. It has taken time to realize the importance of this problem; it was so easily passed over by those with strong beliefs in heredity. Burt quotes Karl Pearson's explanation: "It is not so much that the slums create the dullards, but rather that the duller stocks gravitate automatically to the slums." Growing knowledge of the lifelong effects of early childhood experience and more sophisticated notions of genetic heterogeneity now give the slums more credit for creating dullards than Pearson was willing to concede.

Vernon considers the importance, and the current ignorance, of the specific effects of child-rearing customs and methods. The opportunity and motivation for intellectual development in a child born into a home marked by ambition, school orientation, cultural and intellectual interests, and eagerness to help the child explore ideas and sensory experiences or try out and improve his skills, differ so tremendously from the opportunity and motivation of a child born into a home in which these positive factors are all lacking that the two youngsters start off on completely different roads toward maturity.

We know too little about the specific effects of different child-rearing customs, as Vernon points out, and as Wolfle emphasizes in describing Strodtbeck's comparison of equally bright boys in Jewish and Italian families in the United States. As we acquire more knowledge concerning the specific effects of early childhood differences, we can expect to learn how to develop more high talent, how to develop more talent of moderate levels, and also how to avoid some of the talent loss we now suffer.

The strategy of talent development is Wolfle's theme. Agreeing with Stalnaker, Ghiselli, MacKinnon, and others that the selection of students for promotion to higher levels should take into consideration variables other than the easily and customarily measured ones—school grades and intelligence-test scores—and agreeing with Paterson and Vernon on the need to study the social and cultural factors that stimulate or retard intellectual development, he emphasizes the importance of intellectual diversity and tries to outline a socially useful strategy for talent development. That such a strategy can be presented only in bare and tentative outline reflects the fact stressed by a number of the lecturers that there are large gaps in our knowledge. Much has been learned about the nature of human ability and about how it develops. But there is much that is still unknown.

### *Retrospect*

Walter Van Dyke Bingham, pioneer American applied psychologist, who gave none of these lectures, was responsible for all of them. In his autobiography, Bingham describes one of his major interests as "finding the talented, encouraging their advancement, making known their potentialities."[1] He worked at this self-assigned task consciously, deliberately, and effectively. As he anticipated the end of his own life, this dominant purpose, sup-

1. Walter Van Dyke Bingham, *A History of Psychology in Autobiography,* Vol. IV, pp. 1–26, Clark University Press, Worcester, Mass., 1952.

ported by "a fondness for looking ahead, planning, and *initiating a cooperative enterprise,*"[2] led him to propose the "Discovery of the Talented" project. With his will, he left a memorandum expressing the wish that an annual series of lectures might be established to "rivet attention . . . on the great value of accurate identification of exceptionally promising young people" and also to honor those persons who had made significant contributions to the improvement of methods for the discovery and development of talent. The generosity of his wife, Millicent Todd Bingham, and the cooperation of the American Psychological Association made it possible to carry out that wish. Through 12 lectures, including the one Thurstone was unable to deliver, the "Discovery of the Talented" project continued, each year with a different lecturer, and each year at a different university, a university selected because it had been the site of notable work on talent identification or development. This first phase of the carrying out of Bingham's wish is now ended. Mrs. Bingham has provided for its continuation, however. From now on, the lectures, under the new name of the Walter Van Dyke Bingham Lectures, will be sponsored by and presented at Carnegie-Mellon University—the new name of the Carnegie Institute of Technology, where Dr. Bingham founded the first American department of applied psychology and where his papers and memorabilia are preserved.

Now, more than fifteen years after Dr. Bingham's death, how does the idea seem? The answer was given in part by one of the critics who read the lectures when Harvard University Press was considering bringing them together in book form. He wrote:

> The lectures represent a wide-ranging presentation of a number of current ideas concerning talent by persons who have been closely concerned with research on that topic.

*Ibid.*

> These papers are written in a way which should make the content accessible to a broad audience of interested persons extending well beyond the category of professional psychologists . . . for example, to persons concerned with all aspects of education, with business, with government, and with the arts.

In a larger sense the lectures have been part of a great national and international effort to develop more fully the potentialities of able young people. Private foundations, industry, state governments, and particularly the Federal Government provide vast sums to improve education and to assist students. Special efforts are being made to discover young people whose high potential would otherwise remain hidden. Studies of creativity and other types of accomplishment are vigorously pursued. John Gardner's phrase "the pursuit of excellence" has been so widely used that it has become a cliché. It is neither possible nor worthwhile to determine how much the Discovery of the Talented project contributed to this upsurge of interest in the identification and education of talented young persons. The significant fact is the upsurge itself.

At the same time, there has come to be widespread recognition of the huge social loss we suffer in all ranges of the ability distribution. Far too many children are born into homes that give them little intellectual stimulation, in which their potentialities cannot mature, in which attitudes and customs are so rigid that originality and creativeness cannot flourish, in which the traits and abilities required for effective participation in a complex technological society have little chance to develop. The stultifying effect of these early handicaps on the whole course of life are being realized as never before, and so is their social cost in poverty, apathy, delinquency, crime, inability to compete for jobs in a technological society, and the probability that the unsuccessful will pass on to their children their own frustration, alienation, and what the anthropologist Oscar Lewis has called the "culture of poverty."

Compassion for the individuals who are so trapped, and concern for the health of the society of which they are a part, have now led to the beginnings of massive efforts to remedy the handicaps of a deficient home environment, to overcome the cancer of poverty, and to raise the deprived closer to the level of the average in education, marketable abilities, and self-esteem. These efforts are mandatory, for to the extent that they succeed, they will raise the whole tone and level of accomplishment of society as well as the level of satisfaction and well-being of its members.

But by themselves, these efforts are not enough. Herbert J. Muller, philosophizing on what makes a civilization succeed or fail, concluded that the most reasonable ideal is a democratic society in which there is "culture and education for all, within their capacity." But he went on to remind us that achievement of this ideal requires special attention to those who can contribute most.

> The creative achievements of civilization to date have been primarily the work of an elite, and the greatest achievements will always be due immediately to the gifted few. Ideally, democracy would mean not merely a general rise in the culture of the masses but an elite that is freely recruited, that may be enlarged and constantly invigorated by special talent from the ranks. . . .
>
> For us, the last word is a challenge to the educated, privileged classes. The problem today is not merely a matter of improving the minds and tastes of common men. It is also a question of whether the elite can provide better political, intellectual, and spiritual leadership than it has in all previous societies. For if the creative achievements of civiliza-

> tion have been due primarily to the elite, so too have the failures of civilization.[3]

"Finding the talented, encouraging their advancement, making known their potentialities" will continue to serve two high purposes: gifted individuals will be helped to fulfill their promise and civilization will be enriched.

Washington, D.C., October 21, 1968 Dael Wolfle

3. Herbert J. Muller, *The Uses of the Past,* Oxford University Press, Oxford, 1952, and New American Library, New York, 1954.

## *Contents*

*The Discovery of Talent*

*The Walter Van Dyke Bingham Lectures on the Development of Exceptional Abilities and Capacities*

*Lewis M. Terman*

# *The Discovery and Encouragement of Exceptional Talent*[1]

I am deeply sensible of the honor of being invited by the American Psychological Association, through its special committee, to give the initial lecture in the Walter V. Bingham Lectureship series.

I am especially happy that Chancellor Kerr and the psychology department of the University of California graciously acceded to my request that the address be given here, where I have many friends and where so much notable research has been done on the mental, physical, and personality development of children; where such famous experiments have been made on the purposive behavior of rats, both gifted and dull; where authoritarian minds have been so exhaustively probed; and where the recently established Institute of Personality Assessment is engaged in such promising investigations.

Before beginning my lecture I should like to pay tribute to the life work of the late Walter Van Dyke Bingham, at whose request

1. This paper is based on the first Walter Van Dyke Bingham Lecture, given at the University of California at Berkeley, March 25, 1954. It was first published in the *American Psychologist*, 1954, vol. 9, no. 6 (June), pp. 221–230.

this lectureship was established by Mrs. Bingham. Born in Iowa in 1880, young Walter early demonstrated his exceptional gifts by skipping both the third and fourth grades and by graduating from high school at the age of 16. As a freshman in college he was the youngest in his class and the only one to make a straight A record. After graduating from Beloit College he taught in high schools for four years, then entered the graduate school of the University of Chicago and in 1908 won his doctorate in psychology with honors. From 1908 to 1910 he was instructor at Teachers College and assistant to Edward L. Thorndike. In 1910 he was appointed assistant professor at Dartmouth to teach all their classes in psychology, but when he left there five years later the staff included an instructor and two full professors, all selected by Dr. Bingham. His rare ability to recognize exceptional talent is indicated by the fact that both of these professors became college presidents.

From 1915 to 1924 Dr. Bingham was professor of psychology and head of the division of applied psychology at the Carnegie Institute of Technology, and it was here that he found the opportunity he had long wanted to promote large-scale investigations in applied psychology. The faculty he assembled for that purpose was one of the most distinguished ever brought together anywhere in this country. Among them were J. B. Miner, L. L. Thurstone, Walter Dill Scott, Kate Gordon, and E. K. Strong. Three others appointed as consultants were F. L. Wells, G. M. Whipple, and Raymond Dodge. It was this faculty that, under the wise leadership of Dr. Bingham, laid the solid foundation for vocational and industrial psychology in America.

When our country entered the war in 1917, nearly all of the Carnegie group were soon engaged in psychological work either for the Surgeon General or for the War Department or for both. Dr. Bingham was a member of Yerkes' committee of seven that devised the army mental tests, in 1917–18 was a member of the Committee on Classification of Personnel (the committee charged with devising and administering vocational tests in all the army camps), and in 1918–19 was Lt. Colonel in the Personnel Branch of the Army General Staff.

During World War II even greater service was rendered by Dr. Bingham as chief psychologist for the Office of Adjutant General from 1940 to 1946. In this capacity he and his committee were responsible not only for the Army General Classification Test that was administered to the many millions of inductees, but also for advising on the entire program of psychological services in the armed forces. In this capacity too he was in position to influence the selection of men best qualified to head the various branches of military psychology. I have no doubt that the extraordinary success of the work accomplished by psychologists during the war was largely due to his leadership and to his judgment of men.

If time permitted, I should like to tell you about his more than 200 publications, about the great variety of problems they dealt with, and the contributions they made in several fields of psychology, but I am sure that if Dr. Bingham were here he would want me to get on with our scheduled program.

I have often been asked how I happened to become interested in mental tests and gifted children. My first introduction to the scientific problems posed by intellectual differences occurred well over a half-century ago when I was a senior in psychology at Indiana University and was asked to prepare two reports for a seminar, one on mental deficiency and one on genius. Up to that time, despite the fact that I had graduated from a normal college as a Bachelor of Pedagogy and had taught school for five years, I had never so much as heard of a mental test. The reading for those two reports opened up a new world to me, the world of Galton, Binet, and their contemporaries. The following year my MA thesis on leadership among children (Terman, 1904) was based in part on tests used by Binet in his studies of suggestibility.

Then I entered Clark University, where I spent considerable time during the first year in reading on mental tests and precocious children. Child prodigies, I soon learned, were at that time in bad repute because of the prevailing belief that they were usually psychotic or otherwise abnormal and almost sure to burn themselves out quickly or to develop postadolescent stupidity. "Early ripe, early rot" was a slogan frequently encountered. By the time I reached my last graduate year, I decided to find out for myself how precocious children differ from the mentally backward, and accordingly chose as my doctoral dissertation an experimental study of the intellectual processes of fourteen boys, seven of them picked as the brightest and seven as the dullest in a large city school (Terman, 1906). These subjects I put through a great variety of intelligence tests, some of them borrowed from Binet and others, many of them new. The tests were given individually and required a total of 40 or 50 hours for each subject. The experiment contributed little or nothing to science, but it contributed a lot to my future thinking. Besides "selling" me completely on the value of mental tests as a research method, it offered an ideal escape from the kinds of laboratory work which I disliked and in which I was more than ordinarily inept. (Edward Thorndike confessed to me once that *his* lack of mechanical skill was partly responsible for turning *him* to mental tests and to the kinds of experiments on learning that required no apparatus.)

However, it was not until I got to Stanford in 1910 that I was able to pick up with mental tests where I had left off at Clark University. By that time Binet's 1905 and 1908 scales had been published, and the first thing I undertook at Stanford was a tentative revision of his 1908 scale. This, after further revisions, was published in 1916. The standardization of the scale was based on tests of a thousand children whose IQ's ranged from 60 to 145. The contrast in intellectual performance between the dullest and the brightest of a given age so intensified my earlier interest in the gifted that I decided to launch an ambitious study of such children at the earliest opportunity.

My dream was realized in the spring of 1921 when I obtained a generous grant from the Commonwealth Fund of New York City for the purpose of locating a thousand subjects of IQ 140 or higher. More than that number were selected by Stanford-Binet tests from the kindergarten through the eighth grade, and a group mental test given in 95 high schools provided nearly 400 additional subjects. The latter, plus those I had located before 1921, brought the number close to 1,500. The average IQ was approximately 150, and 80 were 170 or higher (Terman, 1925).

The twofold purpose of the project was, first of all, to find what traits characterize children of high IQ, and secondly, to follow them for as many years as possible to see what kind of adults they might become. This meant that it was necessary to select a group representative of high-testing children in general. With the help of four field assistants, we canvassed a school population of nearly a quarter million in the urban and semiurban areas of California. Two careful checks on the methods used showed that not more than 10 or 12 percent of the children who could have qualified for the group in the schools canvassed were missed. A sample of close to 90 percent insured that whatever traits were typical of these children would be typical of high-testing children in any comparable school population.

Time does not permit me to describe the physical measurements, medical examinations, achievement tests, character and interest tests, or the trait ratings and other supplementary information obtained from parents and teachers. Nor can I here describe the comparative data we obtained for control groups of unselected children. The more important results, however, can be stated briefly: children of IQ 140 or higher are, in general, appreciably superior to unselected children in physique, health, and social adjustment; markedly superior in moral attitudes as measured either by character tests or by trait ratings; and vastly superior in their mastery of school subjects as shown by a three-hour battery of achievement tests. In fact, the typical child of the group had mastered the school subjects to a point about two grades beyond the one in which he was enrolled, some of them three or four grades beyond. Moreover, his ability as evidenced by achievement in the different school subjects is so general as to refute completely the traditional belief that gifted children are usually one-sided. I take some pride in the fact that not one of the major conclusions we drew in the early 1920's regarding the traits that are typical of gifted children has been overthrown in the three decades since then.

Results of thirty years' follow-up of these subjects by field studies in 1927–28, 1939–40, and 1951–52, and by mail follow-up at other dates, show that the incidence of mortality, ill health, insanity, and alcoholism is in each case below that for the generality of corresponding age, that the great majority are still well adjusted socially, and that the delinquency rate is but a fraction of what it is in the general population. Two forms of our difficult Concept Mastery Test, devised especially to reach into the stratosphere of adult intelligence, have been administered to all members of the group who could be visited by the field assistants, including some 950 tested in 1939–40 and more than 1,000 in 1951–52. On both tests they scored on the average about as far above the generality of adults as they had scored above the generality of children when we selected them. Moreover, as Dr. Bayley and Mrs. Oden have shown, in the twelve-year interval between the two tests, 90 percent increased their intellectual stature as measured by this test. "Early ripe, early rot" simply does not hold for these subjects. So far, no one has developed postadolescent stupidity!

As for schooling, close to 90 percent entered college and 70 percent graduated. Of those graduating, 30 percent were awarded honors and about two-thirds remained for graduate work. The educational record would have been still better but for the fact that a majority reached college age during the great depression. In their undergraduate years 40 percent of the men and 20 percent of the women earned half or more of their college expenses, and the total of undergraduate and graduate expenses earned amounted to $670,000, not counting stipends from scholarships and fellowships, which amounted to $350,000.

The cooperation of the subjects is indicated by the fact that we have been able to keep track of more than 98 percent of the original group, thanks to the rapport fostered by the incomparable field and office assistants I have had from the beginning of the study to the present. I dislike to think how differently things could have gone with helpers even a little less competent.

The achievement of the group to midlife is best illustrated by the case histories of the 800 men, since only a minority of the women have gone out for professional careers (Terman, 1954). By 1950, when the men had an average age of 40 years, they had published 67 books (including 46 in the fields of science, arts, and the humanities, and 21 books of fiction). They had published more than 1,400 scientific, technical, and professional articles; over 200 short stories, novelettes, and plays; and 236 miscellaneous articles on a great variety of subjects. They had also authored more than 150 patents. The figures on publications do not include the hundreds of publications by journalists that classify as news stories; editorials, or newspaper columns; nor do they include the hundreds if not thousands of radio and TV scripts.

The 800 men include 78 who have taken a PhD degree or its equivalent, 48 with a medical degree, 85 with a law degree, 74 who are teaching or have taught in a four-year college or university, 51 who have done basic research in the physical sciences or engineering, and 104 who are engineers but have done only applied research or none. Of the scientists, 47 are listed in the

1949 edition of *American Men of Science.* Nearly all of these numbers are from 10 to 20 or 30 times as large as would be found for 800 men of corresponding age picked at random in the general population, and are sufficient answer to those who belittle the significance of IQ differences.

The follow-up of these gifted subjects has proved beyond question that tests of "general intelligence," given as early as six, eight, or ten years, tell a great deal about the ability to achieve either presently or 30 years hence. Such tests do not, however, enable us to predict what direction the achievement will take, and least of all do they tell us what personality factors or what accidents of fortune will affect the fruition of exceptional ability. Granting that both interest patterns and special aptitudes play important roles in the making of a gifted scientist, mathematician, mechanic, artist, poet, or musical composer, I am convinced that to achieve greatly in almost any field, the special talents have to be backed up by a lot of Spearman's *g*, by which is meant the kind of general intelligence that requires ability to form many sharply defined concepts, to manipuate them, and to perceive subtle relationships between them; in other words, the ability to engage in abstract thinking.

The study by Catharine Cox of the childhood traits of historical geniuses gives additional evidence regarding the role of general intelligence in exceptional achievement. That study was part of our original plan to investigate superior ability by two methods of approach: (*a*) by identifying and following living gifted subjects from childhood onward; and (*b*) by proceeding in the opposite direction and tracing the mature genius back to his childhood promise. With a second grant from the Commonwealth Fund, the latter approach got under way only a year later than the former and resulted in the magnum opus by Cox entitled *The Early Mental Traits of Three Hundred Geniuses* (1926). Her subjects represented an unbiased selection from the top 510 in Cattell's objectively compiled list of the 1,000 most eminent men of history. Cox and two able assistants then scanned some 3,000 biographies in search of information that would throw light on the early mental development of these subjects. The information thus obtained filled more than 6,000 typed pages. Next, three psychologists familiar with mental age norms read the documentary evidence on all the subjects and estimated for each the IQ that presumably would be necessary to account for the intellectual behavior recorded for given chronological ages. Average of the three IQ estimates was used as the index of intelligence. In fact two IQ's were estimated for each subject, one based on the evidence to age 17, and the other on evidence to the mid-twenties. The recorded evidence on development to age 17 varied from very little to an amount that yielded about as valid an IQ as a good intelligence test would give. Examples of the latter are Goethe, John Stuart Mill, and Francis Galton. It was the documentary information on Galton, which I summarized and published in 1917 (Terman, 1917), that decided me to prepare plans for the kind of study that was carried out by Cox. The average of estimated IQ's for her 300 geniuses was 155, with many going as high as 175 and several as high as 200. Estimates below 120 occurred only when there was little biographical evidence about the early years.

It is easy to scoff at these post-mortem IQ's, but as one of the three psychologists who examined the evidence and made the IQ ratings, I think the author's main conclusion is fully warranted; namely, that "the genius who achieves highest eminence is one whom intelligence tests would have identified as gifted in childhood."

Special attention was given the geniuses who had sometime or other been labeled as backward in childhood, and in every one of these cases the facts clearly contradicted the legend. One of them was Oliver Goldsmith, of whom his childhood teacher is said to have said "Never was so dull a boy." The fact is that little Oliver was writing clever verse at 7 years and at 8 was reading Ovid and Horace. Another was Sir Walter Scott, who at 7 not only read widely in poetry but was using correctly in his written prose such words as "melancholy" and "exotic." Other alleged childhood dullards included a number who disliked the usual diet of Latin and Greek but had a natural talent for science. Among these were the celebrated German chemist Justus von Liebig, the great English anatomist John Hunter, and the naturalist Alexander von Humboldt, whose name is scattered so widely over the maps of the world.

In the cases just cited one notes a tendency for the direction of later achievement to be foreshadowed by the interests and preoccupations of childhood. I have tried to determine how frequently this was true of the 100 subjects in Cox's group whose childhood was best documented. Very marked foreshadowing was noted in the case of more than half of the group, none at all in less than a fourth. Macaulay, for example, began his career as historian at the age of 6 with what he called a "Compendium of Universal History," filling a quire of paper before he lost interest in the project. Ben Franklin before the age of 17 had displayed nearly all the traits that characterized him in middle life: scientific curiosity, religious heterodoxy, wit and buffoonery, political and business shrewdness, and ability to write. At 11 Pascal was so interested in mathematics that his father thought it best to deprive him of books on this subject until he had first mastered Latin and Greek. Pascal secretly proceeded to construct a geometry of his own and covered the ground as far as the 32nd proposition of Euclid. His father then relented. At 14 Leibnitz was writing on logic and philosophy and composing what he called "An Alphabet of Human Thought." He relates that at this age he took a walk one afternoon to consider whether he should accept the "doctrine of substantial forms."

Similar foreshadowing is disclosed by the case histories of my gifted subjects. A recent study of the scientists and nonscientists among our 800 gifted men (Terman and Oden, 1947) showed many highly significant differences between the early interests and social attitudes of those who became physical scientists and those who majored in the social sciences, law, or the humanities. Those in medical or biological sciences usually rated on such variables somewhere between the physical scientists and the nonscientists.

What I especially want to emphasize, however, is that both the evidence on early mental development of historical geniuses and that obtained by follow-up of gifted subjects selected in childhood by mental tests point to the conclusion that capacity to achieve far beyond the average can be detected early in life by a well-constructed ability test that is heavily weighted with the g factor. It remains to be seen how much the prediction of future achievement can be made more specific as to field by getting, in addition, measures of ability factors that are largely independent of g. It would seem that a 20-year follow-up of the thousands of school children who have been given Thurstone's test of seven "primary mental abilities" would help to provide the answer. At present the factor analysts don't agree on how many "primary" mental abilities there are, nor exactly on what they are. The experts in this field are divided into two schools. The British school, represented by Thomson, Vernon, and Burt, usually stop with the identification of at most three or four group factors in addition to g, while some representing the American school feed the scores of 40 or 50 kinds of tests into a hopper and manage to extract from them what they believe to be a dozen or fifteen separate factors. Members of the British school are as a rule very skeptical about the realities underlying the minor group factors. There are also American psychologists, highly skilled in psychometrics, who share this skepticism. It is to be hoped that further research will give us more information than we now have about the predictive value of the group factors. Until such information is available, the scores on group factors can contribute little to vocational guidance beyond what a good test of general intelligence will provide.

I have always stressed the importance of *early* discovery of exceptional abilities. Its importance is now highlighted by the facts Harvey Lehman has disclosed in his monumental studies of the relation between age and creative achievement (Lehman, 1953). The striking thing about his age curves is how early in life the period of maximum creativity is reached. In nearly all fields of science, the best work is done between ages 25 and 35, and rarely later than 40. The peak productivity for works of lesser merit is usually reached 5 to 10 years later; this is true in some twenty fields of science, in philosophy, in most kinds of musical composition, in art, and in literature of many varieties. The lesson for us from Lehman's statistics is that the youth of high achievement potential should be well trained for his life work before too many of his most creative years have been passed.

This raises the issue of educational acceleration for the gifted. It seems that the schools are more opposed to acceleration now than they were thirty years ago. The lockstep seems to have become more and more the fashion, notwithstanding the fact that practically everyone who has investigated the subject is against it. Of my gifted group, 29 percent managed to graduate from high school before the age of 16½ years (62 of these before 15½), but I doubt if so many would be allowed to do so now. The other 71 percent graduated between 16½ and 18½. We have compared the accelerated with the nonaccelerated on numerous case-history variables. The two groups differed very little in childhood IQ, their health records are equally good, and as adults they are equally well adjusted socially. More of the accelerates graduated from college, and on the average nearly a year and a half earlier than the nonaccelerates; they averaged higher in college grades and more often remained for graduate work. Moreover, the accelerates on the average married .7 of a year earlier, have a trifle lower divorce rate, and score just a little higher on a test of marital happiness (Terman and Oden, 1947). So far as college records of accelerates and nonaccelerates are concerned, our data closely parallel those obtained by the late Noel Keys (1938) at the University of California and those by Pressey (Pressey, 1949) and his associates at Ohio State University.

The Ford Fund for the Advancement of Education has awarded annually since 1951 some 400 college scholarships to gifted students who are not over 16½ years old, are a year or even two years short of high school graduation, but show good evidence of ability to do college work. Three quarters of them are between 15½ and 16½ at the time of college entrance. A dozen colleges and universities accept these students and are keeping close track of their success. A summary of their records for the first year shows that they not only get higher grades than their classmates, who average about two years older, but that they are also equally well adjusted socially and participate in as many extracurricular activities (1953). The main problem the boys have is in finding girls to date who are not too old for them! Some of them have started a campaign to remedy the situation by urging that more of these scholarships be awarded to girls.

The facts I have given do not mean that all gifted children should be rushed through school just as rapidly as possible. If that were done, a majority with IQ of 140 could graduate from high school before the age of 15. I do believe, however, that such children should be promoted rapidly enough to permit college entrance by the age of 17 at latest, and that a majority would be better off to enter at 16. The exceptionally bright student who is kept with his age group finds little to challenge his intelligence and all too often develops habits of laziness that later wreck his college career. I could give you some choice examples of this in my gifted group. In the case of a college student who is preparing for a profession in science, medicine, law, or any field of advanced scholarship, graduation at 20 instead of the usual 22 means two years added to his professional career; or the two years saved could be used for additional training beyond the doctorate, if that were deemed preferable.

Learned and Wood (1938) have shown by objective achievement tests in some 40 Pennsylvania colleges how little correlation there is between the student's knowledge and the number of months or years of his college attendance. They found some beginning sophomores who had acquired more knowledge than some seniors near their graduation. They found similarly low correlations between the number of course units a student had in a given field and the amount he knew in that field. Some with only one year of Latin had learned more than others with three years. And, believe it or not, they even found boys just graduating from high school who had more knowledge of science than some college seniors who had majored in science and were about to begin teaching science in high schools! The sensible thing to do, it seems, would be to quit crediting the individual high school or the individual college and begin crediting the individual student. That, essentially, is what the Ford Fund scholarships are intended to encourage.

Instruments that permit the identification of gifted subjects are available in great variety and at nearly all levels from the primary grades to the graduate schools in universities. My rough guess is that at the present time tests of achievement in the school subjects are being given in this country to children below high school at a rate of perhaps ten or twelve million a year, and to high school students another million or two. In addition, perhaps two million tests of intelligence are given annually in the elementary and high schools. The testing of college students began in a small way only 30 years ago; now almost every college in the country requires applicants for admission to take some kind of aptitude test. This is usually a test of general aptitude, but subject-matter tests and tests of special aptitudes are sometimes given to supplement the tests of general aptitude.

The testing movement has also spread rapidly in other countries, especially in Britain and the Commonwealth countries. Godfrey Thomson devised what is now called the Moray House test of intelligence in 1921 to aid in selecting the more gifted 11-year-olds in the primary schools for the privilege of free secondary education. This test has been revised and is given annually to about a half million scholarship candidates. The Moray House tests now include tests of English, arithmetic, and history. In 1932 the Scottish Council for Research in Education (1933) arranged to give the Moray House test of intelligence (a group test) to all the 90,000 children in Scotland who were born in 1921, and actually tested some 87,000 of them. The Stanford-Binet tests have been translated and adapted for use in nearly all the countries of Europe and in several countries of Asia and Latin America. Behind the Iron Curtain, however, mental tests are now banned.

I have discussed only tests of intelligence and of school achievement. There is time to mention only a few of the many kinds of personality tests that have been developed during the last thirty-five years: personality inventories, projective techniques by the dozen, attitude scales by the hundred, interest tests, tests of psychotic and predelinquent tendencies, tests of leadership, marital aptitude, masculinity-femininity, et cetera. The current output of research on personality tests probably equals or exceeds that on intelligence and achievement tests, and is even more exciting.

Along with the increasing use of tests, and perhaps largely as a result of it, there is a growing interest, both here and abroad, in improving educational methods for the gifted. Acceleration of a year or two or three, however desirable, is but a fraction of what is needed to keep the gifted child or youth working at his intellectual best. The method most often advocated is curriculum enrichment for the gifted without segregating them from the ordinary class. Under ideal conditions enrichment can accomplish much, but in these days of crowded schools, when so many teachers are overworked, underpaid, and inadequately trained, curriculum enrichment for a few gifted in a large mixed class cannot begin to solve the problem. The best survey of thought and action in this field of education is the book entitled *The Gifted Child,* written by many authors and published in 1951 (Witty, 1951). In planning for and sponsoring this book, The American Association for Gifted Children has rendered a great service to education.

But however efficient our tests may be in discovering exceptional talents, and whatever the schools may do to foster those discovered, it is the prevailing *Zeitgeist* that will decide, by the rewards it gives or withholds, what talents will come to flower. In Western Europe of the Middle Ages, the favored talents were those that served the Church by providing its priests, the architects of its cathedrals, and the painters of religious themes. A few centuries later the same countries had a renaissance that included science and literature as well as the arts. Although presumably there are as many potential composers of great music as there ever were, and as many potentially great artists as in the days of Leonardo da Vinci and Michelangelo, I am reliably informed that in this country today it is almost impossible for a composer of *serious* music to earn his living except by teaching, and that the situation is much the same, though somewhat less critical, with respect to artists.

The talents most favored by the current *Zeitgeist* are those that can contribute to science and technology. If intelligence and achievement tests don't discover the potential scientist, there is a good chance that the annual Science Talent Search will, though not until the high school years. Since Westinghouse inaugurated in 1942 this annual search for the high school seniors most likely to become creative scientists, nearly 4,000 boys and girls have been picked for honors by Science Service out of the many thousands who have competed. As a result, "Science Clubs of America" now number 15,000 with a third of a million members —a twenty fold increase in a dozen years (Davis, 1953). As our need for more and better scientists is real and urgent, one can rejoice at what the talent search and the science clubs are accomplishing. One may regret, however, that the spirit of the times is not equally favorable to the discovery and encouragement of potential poets, prose writers, artists, statesmen, and social leaders.

But in addition to the over-all climates that reflect the *Zeitgeist,* there are localized climates that favor or hinder the encouragement of given talents in particular colleges and universities. I have in mind especially two recent investigations of the differences among colleges in the later achievement of their graduates. One by Knapp and Goodrich (1952) dealt with the undergraduate origin of 18,000 scientists who got the bachelor's degree between 1924 and 1934 and were listed in the 1944 edition of *American Men of Science.* The list of 18,000 was composed chiefly of men who had taken a PhD degree, but included a few without a PhD who were starred scientists. The IBM cards for these men were then sorted according to the college from which they obtained the bachelor's degree, and an index of productivity was computed for each college in terms of the proportion of its male graduates who were in the list of 18,000. Some of the results were surprising, not to say sensational. The institutions that were most productive of future scientists between 1924 and 1934 were not the great universities, but the small liberal arts colleges. Reed College topped the list with an index of 132 per thousand male graduates. The California Institute of Technology was second with an index of 70. Kalamazoo College was third with 66, Earlham fourth with 57, and Oberlin fifth with 56. Only a half-dozen of the great universities were in the top fifty with a productivity index of 25 or more.

The second study referred to was by Knapp and Greenbaum (1953), who rated educational institutions according to the proportion of their graduates who received certain awards at the graduate level in the six-year period from 1946 to 1951. Three kinds of awards were considered: a PhD degree, a graduate scholarship or fellowship paying at least $400 a year, or a prize at the graduate level won in open competition. The roster of awardees they compiled included 7,000 students who had graduated from 377 colleges and universities. This study differs from the former in three respects: (*a*) it deals with recent graduates, who had not had time to become distinguished but who could be regarded as good bets for the future; (*b*) these good bets were classified according to whether the major field was science, social science, or the humanities; and (*c*) data were obtained for both sexes, though what I shall report here relates only to men. In this study the great universities make a better showing than in the other, but still only a dozen of them are in the top fifty institutions in the production of men who are good bets. In the top ten, the University of Chicago is third, Princeton is eighth, and Harvard is tenth; the other seven in order of rank are Swarthmore 1, Reed 2, Oberlin 4, Haverford 5, California Institute of Technology 6, Carleton 7, and Antioch 9. When the schools were listed separately for production of men who were good bets in science, social science, and the humanities, there were eight that rated in the top twenty on all three lists. These were Swarthmore, Reed, Chicago, Harvard, Oberlin, Antioch, Carleton, and Princeton.

The causes of these differences are not entirely clear. Scores on aptitude tests show that the intelligence of students in a given institution is by no means the sole factor, though it is an important one. Other important factors are the quality of the school's intellectual climate, the proportion of able and inspiring teachers on its faculty, and the amount of conscious effort that is made not only to discover but also to motivate the most highly gifted. The influence of motivation can hardly be exaggerated.

In this address I have twice alluded to the fact that achievement in school is influenced by many things other than the sum total of intellectual abilities. The same is true of success in life. In closing I will tell you briefly about an attempt we made a dozen years ago to identify some of the nonintellectual factors that have influenced life success among the men in my gifted group. Three judges, working independently, examined the records (to 1940) of the 730 men who were then 25 years old or older, and rated each on life success. The criterion of "success" was the extent to which a subject had made use of his superior intellectual ability, little weight being given to earned income. The 150 men rated highest for success and the 150 rated lowest were then compared on some 200 items of information obtained from childhood onward (Terman and Oden, 1947). How did the two groups differ?

During the elementary school years, the A's and C's (as we call them) were almost equally successful. The average grades were about the same, and average scores on achievement tests were only a trifle higher for the A's. Early in high school the groups began to draw apart in scholarship, and by the end of high school the slump of the C's was quite marked. The slump could not be blamed on extracurricular activities, for these were almost twice as common among the A's. Nor was much of it due to difference in intelligence. Although the A's tested on the average a little higher than the C's both in 1922 and 1940, the average score made by the C's in 1940 was high enough to permit brilliant college work, in fact was equaled by only 15 percent of our highly selected Stanford students. Of the A's, 97 percent entered college and 90 percent graduated; of the C's, 68 percent entered but only 37 percent graduated. Of those who graduated, 52 percent of the A's but only 14 percent of the C's graduated with honors. The A's were also more accelerated in school; on the average they were six months younger on completing the eighth grade, 10 months younger at high school graduation, and 15 months younger at graduation from college.

The differences between the educational histories of the A's and C's reflect to some degree the differences in their family backgrounds. Half of the A fathers but only 15 percent of the C fathers were college graduates, and twice as many of A siblings as of C siblings graduated. The estimated number of books in the A homes was nearly 50 percent greater than in the C homes. As of 1928, when the average age of the subjects was about 16 years, more than twice as many of the C parents as of A parents had been divorced.

Interesting differences between the groups were found in the childhood data on emotional stability, social adjustments, and various traits of personality. Of the 25 traits on which each child was rated by parent and teacher in 1922 (18 years before the A and C groups were made up), the only trait on which the C's averaged as high as the A's was general health. The superiority of the A's was especially marked in four volitional traits: prudence, self-confidence, perseverance, and desire to excel. The A's also rated significantly higher in 1922 on leadership, popularity, and sensitiveness to approval or disapproval. By 1940 the difference betwen the groups in social adjustment and all-round mental stability had greatly increased and showed itself in many ways. By that time four-fifths of the A's had married, but only two-thirds of the C's, and the divorce rate for those who had married was twice as high for the C's as for the A's. Moreover, the A's made better marriages; their wives on the average came from better homes, were better educated, and scored higher on intelligence tests.

But the most spectacular differences between the two groups came from three sets of ratings, made in 1940, on a dozen personality traits. Each man rated himself on all the traits, was rated on them by his wife if he had a wife, and by a parent if a parent was still living. Although the three sets of ratings were made independently, they agreed unanimously on the four traits in which the A and C groups differed most widely. These were "persistence in the accomplishment of ends," "integration toward goals, as contrasted with drifting," "self-confidence," and "freedom from inferiority feelings." For each trait three critical ratios were computed showing, respectively, the reliability of the A–C differences in average of self-ratings, ratings by wives, and ratings by parents. The average of the three critical ratios was 5.5 for perseverance, 5.6 for integration toward goals, 3.7 for self-confidence, and 3.1 for freedom from inferiority feelings. These closely parallel the traits that Cox found to be especially characteristic of the 100 leading geniuses in her group whom she rated on many aspects of personality; their three outstanding traits she defined as "persistence of motive and effort," "confidence in their abilities," and "strength or force of character."

There was one trait on which only the parents of our A and C men were asked to rate them; that trait was designated "common sense." As judged by parents, the A's are again reliably superior, the A–C difference in average rating having a critical ratio of 3.9. We are still wondering what self-ratings by the subjects and ratings of them by their wives on common sense would have shown if we had been impudent enough to ask for them!

Everything considered, there is nothing in which our A and C groups present a greater contrast than in drive to achieve and in all-round mental and social adjustment. Our data do not support the theory of Lange-Eichbaum (1932) that great achievement usually stems from emotional tensions that border on the abnormal. In our gifted group, success is associated with stability rather than instability, with absence rather than with presence of disturbing conflicts—in short with well-balanced temperament and with freedom from excessive frustrations. The Lange-Eichbaum theory may explain a Hitler, but hardly a Churchill; the junior senator from Wisconsin, possibly, but not a Jefferson or a Washington.

At any rate, we have seen that intellect and achievement are far from perfectly correlated. To identify the internal and external factors that help or hinder the fruition of exceptional talent, and to measure the extent of their influences, are surely among the major problems of our time. These problems are not new: their existence has been recognized by countless men from Plato to Francis Galton. What is new is the general awareness of them caused by the manpower shortage of scientists, engineers, moral leaders, statesmen, scholars, and teachers that the country must have if it is to survive in a threatened world. These problems are now being investigated on a scale never before approached, and by a new generation of workers in several related fields. Within a couple of decades vastly more should be known than we know today about our resources of potential genius, the environmental circumstances that favor its expression, the emotional compulsions that give it dynamic quality, and the personality distortions that can make it dangerous.

### *References*

Cox, Catharine C. *The early mental traits of three hundred geniuses.* Vol. II of *Genetic studies of genius,* Terman, L. M. (ed.). Stanford: Stanford Univer. Press, 1926.

Davis, W. Communicating science. *J. atomic Scientists,* 1953, 337–340.

Keys, N. The underage student in high school and college. *Univer. Calif. Publ. Educ.,* 1938, 7, 145–272.

Knapp, R. H., & Goodrich, H. B. *Origins of American scientists.* Chicago: Univer. of Chicago Press, 1952.

Knapp, R. H., & Greenbaum, J. J. *The younger American scholar: his collegiate origins.* Chicago: Univer. of Chicago Press, 1953.

Lange-Eichbaum, W. *The problem of genius.* New York: Macmillan, 1932.

Learned, W. S., & Wood, B. D. The student and his knowledge. *Carnegie Found. Adv. Teaching Bull.*, 1938, No. 29.

Lehman, H. C. *Age and achievement.* Princeton: Princeton Univer. Press, 1953.

Pressey, S. L. *Educational acceleration: appraisals and basic problems.* Columbus: Ohio State Univer. Press, 1949.

Terman, L. M. A preliminary study in the psychology and pedagogy of leadership. *Pedag. Sem.*, 1904, *11*, 413–451.

Terman, L. M. Genius and stupidity: a study of some of the intellectual processes of seven "bright" and seven "dull" boys. *Pedag. Sem.*, 1906, *13*, 307–373.

Terman, L. M. The intelligence quotient of Francis Galton in childhood. *Amer. J. Psychol.*, 1917, *28*, 209–215.

Terman, L. M. (ed.), *et al. Mental and physical traits of a thousand gifted children.* Vol. I of *Genetic studies of genius*, Terman, L. M. (ed.). Stanford: Stanford Univer. Press, 1925.

Terman, L. M., & Oden, M. H. *The gifted child grows up.* Vol. IV of *Genetic studies of genius*, Terman, L. M. (ed.). Stanford: Stanford Univer. Press, 1947.

Terman, L. M. Scientists and nonscientists in a group of 800 gifted men. *Psychol. Monogr.*, 1954, Vol. *68*, no. 7, 1–43.

Witty, P. (ed.). *The gifted child.* Boston: Heath, 1951.

*Bridging the gap between school and college.* New York: The Fund for the Advancement of Education, 1953.

*The intelligence of Scottish children.* Scottish Council for Research in Education. London: Univer. of London Press, 1933.

# *Donald G. Paterson* — *The Conservation of Human Talent*[1]

When I began thinking about the subject matter of tonight's lecture, I planned to discuss the interrelation of ability, achievement, vocational interests, and job satisfaction and, especially, the perplexing lack of relationship between measured vocational interests on the one hand and achievement and job satisfaction on the other. Later on, when I decided to discuss the conservation of human talent, I found myself concerned not so much with the technicalities primarily of interest to the vocational and personnel psychologist but rather with an attempt to portray the role of vocational and personnel psychology in a free America. Thus, my intent is to appeal to a wider audience in the hope that, perhaps, my remarks may help to secure a better public understanding of what my professional colleagues are attempting to do. It is my conviction that Walter Bingham would want this type of emphasis just as much as he would approve a talk emphasizing the more technical aspects of our work.

The subtitle of my topic is "The Role of Vocational Psychology

1. This paper is based on the Walter Van Dyke Bingham Lecture given at the Ohio State University, April 17, 1956. It was first published in the *American Psychologist*, 1957, vol. 12, no. 3 (March), pp. 134–144.

in Manpower Management." Perhaps it would be well, at the outset, to provide a few definitions.

We define vocational psychology as the study of the relationship of personality to vocational and occupational adjustment. The term "personality" is used in a broad sense to include abilities, aptitudes, interests, attitudes, and all other personal characteristics. The term "occupational adjustment" refers to the extent to which a person's unique characteristics are in harmony with the short-run and the long-run demands of the vocation or occupation in which he finds himself.

By manpower management we mean the conservation and optimal utilization of our human resources in our total economy. In addition, we emphasize that the idea of manpower management should be broadened to include the idea of manpower self-management. In a free, democratic society, we cannot achieve an optimal utilization of our human resources without recognizing the importance and dignity of the individual and his right to choose freely the occupation for which he feels he is fitted. It is this emphasis that differentiates our task in America from what goes on in a totalitarian state. Here, we assume that the state exists to serve the individual, whereas totalitarianism assumes that the individual exists to serve the state.

My own interest in this topic goes back to my graduate student days here at Ohio State University before World War I. My major advisor—the late Dr. Rudolf Pintner—was busy helping to create a psychology of individual differences by quantitative studies of a wide variety of groups of children and adults. And he had the knack of enlisting the energies of his students in this exciting quest. He and his students studied the feebleminded, the delinquent, the deaf, the blind, the unemployed. In these studies we used available mental test methods, improved existing tests, and devised new tests. The immediate aim was to get a better understanding of the educational, occupational, and social adjustment problems of children and adults. The ultimate aim, however, was to aid the individual to make better educational, occupational, and social adjustments.

This experience was followed by the great adventure of World War I when we were given the opportunity to apply psychological methods to the solution of military manpower problems. In this work, we learned to work with the medical profession, with the psychiatrists, with personnel managers from business and industry, and with line and staff officers at all levels of authority and responsibility. Here again, we adapted available psychological tests and rating scales, improved existing methods, and devised new methods. The aim, of course, was to aid our armed forces to utilize the talents of our civilian-soldiers with a minimum of waste in time and in manpower. The slogan behind all of this effort became "the right man in the right place."

Following World War I, great efforts were made to apply this experience to business and industry and to education. We witnessed the slow growth of vocational psychology and personnel administration during the 1920's. Then came the depression of the 1930's. With it came an accelerated attack on problems of employment, unemployment, and relief. I refer to the work of the Minnesota Employment Stabilization Research Institute in the early 1930's followed by the Adjustment Service in New York City which put on a one-year demonstration of the values of the vocational and avocational counseling of some 12,000 unemployed persons. Then came the Occupational Research Program of the United States Employment Service most ably directed by Drs. W. H. Stead, M. R. Trabue, and C. L. Shartle. This enterprise resulted in an improved public employment service with testing and counseling services available in the principal cities of the United States. Improved programs for the vocational counseling of the physically handicapped in various states of the union as well as intensive vocational counseling services for our veterans have been introduced on an unprecedented scale. In addition, our more progressive business and industrial organizations have organized more effective employment and personnel departments to improve the selection and placement of men and women in jobs for which they are best fitted.

During the 1930's a similar attack on manpower problems was being made in education. I refer to the work of the American Council on Education and its committees on student personnel work and its work in developing the cooperative testing program now taken over by the Educational Testing Service of Princeton, New Jersey. This has led to state-wide testing programs at the secondary school level, the introduction of student counseling programs in colleges and in high schools, and the attempt of secondary schools and colleges to adjust their curricular offerings to the wide range of individual differences in aptitudes, abilities, and interests found in any representative group of youngsters and adults. In short, all possible efforts are now being made to individualize mass education at every level of education.

I must add that World War II and events since World War II have greatly expanded our efforts in all these directions. And this has been accompanied by increased recognition of the need for improved professional competence of all those who are responsible for aiding each individual to make an optimal educational and occupational adjustment in our increasingly complex world of work. If this objective could be fully attained, the proportion of our population which is properly labeled "occupationally maladjusted" would be held to a minimum.

Time precludes discussion of the multiplicity of causes of occupational maladjustment. I would, however, like to mention widespread discrimination in education and in employment of members of minority groups, of younger workers lacking job experience, of older workers, of women, and of the physically handicapped. In addition, there is, in our culture, the white collar complex, the "hitching your wagon to a star" idea, and the "log cabin to the White House" tradition which leads youth and adults alike to strive for the highest occupational levels regardless of whether or not they possess the necessary aptitudes, abilities, and interests needed for even minimum success at these levels. William Proctor and Helen Ward (1923) of California, in the early 1920's, showed that high school youngsters with IQs below 100 overwhelmingly chose the top occupational levels, whereas a follow-up four years later showed most of them to be in the unskilled and semiskilled levels of work. Details are shown in Table 1. There is no reason to believe that youngsters today are much more realistic or rational in their vocational aspirations. It appears that four-fifths of our youth aspire to high level jobs in which only one-fifth of our labor force is employed. Furthermore, this same type of wishful thinking characterizes adult workers as well.

To a considerable degree, this phenomenon appears to be due to false job values permeating our society. I refer to the prestige hierarchy of occupations which was first established by Counts in 1925. In 1945, in discussing this problem before a group of high

Table 1. Occupational choices of low IQ (80–99) high school pupils.

| Occupational Level | Occupational Choice | Occupation Engaged in Four Years Later |
|---|---|---|
| I Professional | 30% | 0% |
| II Business, Clerical | 26% | 5% |
| III Skilled Trades | 44% | 32% |
| IV Semiskilled | 0% | 35% |
| V Unskilled | 0% | 28% |

school counselors, I presented the data by Counts and was immediately assailed because they were certain that these prestige values had been destroyed by the depression of the 1930's, by experiences during World War II, by the growth of courses in occupational information, and by the introduction of educational and vocational counseling services in the high schools. This led us (Deeg and Paterson, 1947) to duplicate the 1925 study in 1946, with the results shown in Table 2. Surprisingly enough, the results remained substantially the same as shown by a correlation of + .97 between the 1925 rank order and the 1946 rank order. If we really believed in the essential dignity of labor, no matter how menial, and that the welfare of our society is really dependent upon the contributions of workers in every

Table 2. Social status ranks of twenty-five occupations obtained in 1925 and in 1946.

| Occupations | Rank Order 1925 | Rank Order 1946 | Occupations | Rank Order 1925 | Rank Order 1946 |
|---|---|---|---|---|---|
| Banker | 1 | 2.5 | Electrician | 13 | 11 |
| Physician | 2 | 1 | Insurance Salesman | 14 | 10 |
| Lawyer | 3 | 2.5 | Mail Carrier | 15 | 14 |
| Supt. of Schools | 4 | 4 | Carpenter | 16 | 15 |
| Civil Engineer | 5 | 5 | Soldier | 17 | 19 |
| Army Captain | 6 | 6 | Plumber | 18 | 17 |
| Foreign Missionary | 7 | 7 | Motorman | 19 | 18 |
| Elem. School Teacher | 8 | 8 | Barber | 20 | 20 |
| Farmer | 9 | 12 | Truck Driver | 21 | 21.5 |
| Machinist | 10 | 9 | Coal Miner | 22 | 21.5 |
| Traveling Salesman | 11 | 16 | Janitor | 23 | 23 |
| Grocer | 12 | 13 | Hod Carrier | 24 | 24 |
| | | | Ditch Digger | 25 | 25 |

occupational group, the prestige hierarchy of occupations would disappear and each occupation would be ranked as equal to every other occupation. Since this is not so, the vocational counselor is confronted by tremendous resistance to wise occupational choices by innumerable youngsters and adults who seek jobs with high prestige rather than jobs for which they are best fitted.

Another type of evidence pointing to widespread occupational dissatisfaction is provided by surveys which asked the adult worker this question: "If you could go back to the age of eighteen and start life over again, would you choose a different career or occupation?" Roper (1938) made this nationwide survey with the following results: (*a*) 41 percent of the total sample answered "Yes," they would change; (*b*) a slightly larger proportion of men than of women would change; (*c*) a slightly larger proportion of older workers than of younger workers would change; and (*d*) a *much* larger proportion of factory workers than of professional workers would change. This last fact points to an occupational hierarchy of job satisfaction in which so-called higher level jobs have the largest proportion of satisfied workers with a constant increase in the proportion of dissatisfied workers as we descend to the semiskilled and unskilled levels of work.

In 1940, our Research Staff at Minnesota working on problems of employment, unemployment, and relief made an opinion survey of selected occupational groups in St. Paul and, among others, used this same question. The results (Paterson and Stone, 1942) were quite similar, as shown in Table 3. Those who answered "Yes" were then asked: "What occupation or career would you choose?" The results, as shown in Table 4, for the three occupational groups having the largest proportion of "Yes" answers indicated a striking tendency to choose the higher level prestige occupations. This suggests that the same tendency to choose high level occupations as was revealed by Proctor and

Ward for high school youngsters in the early 1920's is manifested by adult workers in the early 1940's. There is no reason to believe that the facts would be much different at the present time.

Table 3. Dissatisfaction with life work.[a]

| Occupational Group | Percent Desiring Change |
|---|---|
| Streetcar Operators | 80 |
| City Firemen | 63 |
| Unemployed | 61 |
| Relief Clients | 60 |
| Clerical Workers | 46 |
| Social Workers | 26 |
| Employers | 19 |
| All Groups | 52 |

[a] Selected Occupational Groups, St. Paul, Minnesota, 1941. $N = 1{,}405$.

Table 4. Type of work preferred by those desiring change of life work.

| Type of Work Preferred | Percentage Choosing Type of Work | | |
|---|---|---|---|
| | Streetcar Operators | City Firemen | Clerical Workers |
| | $N = 162$ | $N = 126$ | $N = 102$ |
| Professional & Executive | 34 | 47 | 82 |
| Clerical & Sales | 5 | 5 | 5 |
| Skilled Trades | 22 | 15 | 0 |
| Semiskilled | 0 | 1 | 0 |
| Unskilled | 0 | 0 | 0 |
| Service | 4 | 8 | 1 |
| Farm Work | 9 | 2 | 1 |
| Don't Know | 26 | 22 | 11 |
| Total | 100 | 100 | 100 |

Another important cause of occupational maladjustment is the failure of our educational system to prepare youngsters adequately and, many times, even minimally, for occupational competition upon entering the labor force. All too frequently youngsters are kept in school until age 16, 17, or 18, or even longer, without being given appropriate vocational training needed for economic competition. This results in a sort of wholesale negative vocational guidance program whereby youngsters drop out of school as failures in our characteristically academic types of education. Many are then forced into the labor market with few positive assets that can be used to classify them properly for available jobs. At this point, business and industry frequently make a fatal mistake in classifying such youngsters as fitted for only the unskilled, semiskilled, or other types of work that require little prejob or on-the-job training. If this be in error, the youngster gets trapped in a vicious employment circle. He acquires job experience and as he moves from employer to employer he is tagged by job labels that merely perpetuate his occupational misclassification. This is because of the widespread practice of classifying applicants for employment primarily on the basis of their work histories.

Clear-cut evidence on this point was obtained by our St. Paul study in 1940–41 of a 10 percent sample of applicants for employment in the local Public Employment Office (Yoder *et al.*, 1948). The busy employment interviewers, at that time, were forced to classify applicants primarily on the basis of work histories and a brief interview. Our research staff, on the contrary, classified these same applicants on the basis of complete case histories that included extensive interviewing covering the entire life history of the individual with especial emphasis on home background, education and training, detailed work histories, claimed interests, attitudes, and motivations, plus the administration of general and special aptitude tests, trade tests, achievement tests, interest tests, personality tests, and, finally, clearance reports from previous schools attended, from previous employers, and from social service agencies. Our research staff classifications were aimed at occupational fields that the applicants could enter immediately or that the applicants could probably succeed in if they secured appropriate pre-employment or on-the-job training. The results, as shown in Table 5, reflect a disturbing lack of agreement between the two sets of primary job classifications (ibid., p. 140). There is perfect agreement for only 100 of the 233 male applicants. Thus, there was agreement in only 43 percent of the cases. What is even more disturbing is the extent of the disagreements among the other 57 percent of the applicants.

One of the outstanding findings is the amount of misclassification that appears in the case of those men who were tagged by the Public Employment Service as "semiskilled" or "unskilled." A total of 122 were so classified. There was agreement between the Employment Service Classification and the Research Staff Classification in only 35, or 29 percent, of these applicants. And, what is more important, a considerable number of these so-called semiskilled and unskilled applicants could function in the labor market as skilled workers, in sales work, in clerical types of work, and, in four instances, the appropriate classification would have placed these individuals at the professional, semiprofessional, or managerial levels of work.

If we assume, for the moment, that the Research Staff classifications are correct and that the Employment Service classifications where there is disagreement are incorrect, it is obvious that here is evidence of a tremendous waste of our manpower resources. In other words, our traditional methods fail to classify men properly for work opportunities, and thus there is a violation of the concept of conservation of talent in our society.

The skeptic, however, may believe that the Research Staff

Table 5. Employment Service primary job classifications of 233 male unemployed registrants compared with Research Institute primary job classifications of the same individuals (1940–41).

| Employment Service Classifications | Research Institute Classifications: Professional, Semiprofessional, and Managerial | Clerical | Sales | Service | Farm | Skilled | Semiskilled | Unskilled | Total |
|---|---|---|---|---|---|---|---|---|---|
| Professional, Semiprofessional, and Managerial | 8 | 4 | 2 | – | – | – | 1 | 1 | 16 |
| Clerical | 1 | 17 | 5 | 1 | – | 2 | 2 | 2 | 30 |
| Sales | 1 | 5 | 4 | – | – | 1 | – | – | 11 |
| Service | – | 1 | – | 7 | 3 | – | 1 | – | 12 |
| Farm | – | – | – | – | – | – | – | – | – |
| Skilled | – | 1 | – | 1 | – | 29 | 7 | 4 | 42 |
| Semiskilled | 2 | 4 | 3 | 2 | 7 | 11 | 27 | 6 | 62 |
| Unskilled | 2 | 7 | 4 | 7 | 10 | 7 | 15 | 8 | 60 |
| Total | 14 | 39 | 18 | 18 | 20 | 50 | 53 | 21 | 233 |

classifications are as likely to be in error as the Employment Service classifications. For evidence on this point, we can point to the accuracy of our Research Staff classifications made on a similar basis in 1932 as revealed by a follow-up study of the occupation engaged in ten years later (ibid., p. 147). The results are presented in Table 6. These 144 adults were tested, classified, and counseled in 1932, and predictions were later made as to the probable type and level of occupational competition to be expected in 1942. There was perfect agreement in 77 percent of the cases, underprediction in 13 percent and overprediction in 10 percent. Analysis of the case records in the 23 percent of disagreements indicates a variety of factors at work, the most important of which seemed to be unusually good or poor motivation or personality and temperamental difficulties.

To go back to the misclassification of "unskilled" workers shown in Table 5, perhaps a case history of one such individual will best dramatize what is involved.

> *Family Background.* Mr. Harolds was one of nine children whose father was a skilled worker in the building trades. The family lived in several small towns. Mr. Harolds graduated from high school in the mid-thirties at age 19.
>
> *Physical Handicap.* Mr. Harolds was unable to enter the labor market for three years after high school graduation because of a bone condition that developed following surgery.
>
> *Rehabilitation Service Experience.* When sufficiently recovered, Mr. Harolds was put in touch with the State Vocational Rehabilitation Service. Because he was a high school graduate, this Service sent him to a business college to take a ten-month secretarial course. But Mr. Harolds could not become interested in this type of course and withdrew after six months.

Table 6. Relation between future occupational group as predicted in 1932 and actual occupational group in 1942.[a]

| Occupational Group as Predicted in 1932 | Actual Occupational Group in 1942: Profes-sional, Scien-tific | Profes-sional, Verbal | Profes-sional, Mana-gerial | Clerical, Skilled | Clerical, Routine | Sales, Per-sonal | Sales, Rou-tine | Mechan-ical, Skilled | Mechan-ical, Unskilled Semi-skilled | Casual | Total |
|---|---|---|---|---|---|---|---|---|---|---|---|
| Professional, scientific | 2 | – | – | – | – | – | – | 1 | – | – | 3 |
| Professional, verbal | – | 3 | 1 | – | – | – | – | – | – | – | 4 |
| Professional, managerial | – | 1 | 2 | – | – | – | – | – | – | – | 3 |
| Clerical, skilled | – | – | 2 | 9 | – | – | 1 | – | – | – | 12 |
| Clerical, routine | – | – | 1 | – | 15 | – | – | 1 | 1 | 2 | 20 |
| Sales, personal | – | 1 | – | – | – | 2 | – | – | – | 1 | 4 |
| Sales, routine | – | – | – | – | – | – | 1 | – | – | – | 1 |
| Mechanical, skilled | – | – | – | 1 | – | – | – | 25 | 1 | – | 27 |
| Mechanical, unskilled, semiskilled | – | – | 2 | – | 2 | 1 | – | 1 | 34 | 6 | 46 |
| Casual | – | – | 1 | – | 1 | – | 1 | – | 3 | 18 | 24 |
| Total | 2 | 5 | 9 | 10 | 18 | 3 | 3 | 28 | 39 | 27 | 144 |

[a] From Farabaugh, Mary. A longitudinal study of vocational adjustment during the depression years. Unpublished doctor's dissertation, University of Minnesota, 1946.

*Work Experience, 1938–1942.* Mr. Harolds entered the labor market in 1938 and held a number of seasonal jobs. These included working as a house painter, farm laborer, surveyor's helper, stock boy and sales worker in a general store, and window washer. He was not interested in any of these jobs, and employer reports reflected this lack of interest. When he applied for work in the St. Paul Public Employment Office in 1942, he was classified as "Unskilled." He happened to turn up in our Employment Research Institute 10 percent sample of applicants.

*Research Staff Classification.* He was classified as fitted for potential "professional levels of work." This classification was based chiefly on the test scores obtained at the time and also on his earlier test and scholastic record at time of high school graduation.

*Test Data. 1. General Ability.* Mr. Harolds made a high score on the Pressey Classification Test—96th percentile on adult norms. His College Ability Test percentile rank at time of high school graduation was 92 and his High School Scholarship Rank was at the 93rd percentile in a graduating class of over 100.

2. *Clerical Ability.* His clerical ability was poor. He was at the 10th and 15th percentiles on the two parts of the Minnesota Clerical Test and in the lowest third on the USES Worker Analysis Section Test of Clerical Ability. Had the Rehabilitation Service tested this man seven years earlier, they probably would not have assigned him to a business college secretarial course.

3. *Dexterities and Mechanical Ability.* No outstanding scores were made on these tests.

4. *Personality Tests.* Scores on the Bell Adjustment Inventory revealed him to be "Very retiring" in the social area and to be somewhat disturbed in the emotional area. He

reported to the vocational counselor that he was discouraged, that he felt he was quite a disappointment to his parents and to himself because he had been out of high school so long without making any real progress. The counselor wrote: "I feel that *if* he can make a satisfactory job adjustment, his personality difficulties will clear up."

5. *Interests.* There were no crystallized vocational interest patterns on Strong's Vocational Interest Blank except for two B+'s in the verbal-linguistic occupations (Lawyer and Author-Journalist).

*Counselor's Judgment.* In view of all ascertained facts concerning Mr. Harolds' family background, failure in clerical training, and poor work history, but with his superior high school record, and superior college ability test scores, the counselor urged him to enter college and attempt to prepare himself for a professional career. The problem was primarily one of motivating him to attempt college work even though he would have to be entirely self-supporting. After many counseling sessions, Mr. Harolds decided to carry out this plan.

*Subsequent Thirteen-Year History.* Mr. Harolds entered the University of Minnesota in September, 1942, and graduated in June, 1946, receiving the BA degree magna cum laude, together with membership in Phi Beta Kappa. He majored in one of the social sciences. He then earned his MA in 1948 and his PhD in 1950 in the same social science. Since then he has made steady progress in the academic world beginning as an Assistant Professor in a midwestern state university.

Our latest report, in December, 1955, indicates continued success and satisfaction with his professional attainments.

*Implications.* Time does not permit adequate discussion of

the implications of the case of Mr. Harolds. The following, however, appear to be worthy of emphasis.

1. In the mid-thirties, there was no adequate program of educational and vocational counseling in the high school attended by Mr. Harolds. No one apparently recognized the high potential of this youngster, at least to the extent of counseling him to prepare for a professional type of work by going to college.

2. In the mid-thirties, rehabilitation work for the physically handicapped was prescientific in the sense that Mr. Harolds was forced into a ten-month secretarial training program without its being realized that he lacked clerical aptitude and measured clerical interests. This action was taken in spite of his own expressed distaste for clerical work. The decision seemed to have been based primarily on the fact that this person was a high school graduate and could be prepared for job competition in a relatively inexpensive ten-month secretarial training program which would also be compatible with his physical handicap. This action proved to be wasteful of taxpayers' funds and only served to embark Mr. Harolds on a program of job failure. This is a case of "penny-wise and pound-foolish."

3. The Public Employment Service in 1942 misclassified Mr. Harolds as an "unskilled laborer" primarily on the basis of his "job-hopping" work history for a period of some four years.

4. The Employment Research Staff, because of its comprehensive testing and interviewing program plus its consulting of school records and of all previous employers, was able to recognize this man's potential assets and to take the necessary steps to translate a record of job marginality and job failure into a record of outstanding achievement at the PhD level of professional training. Here is a concrete example of the kind of vocational counseling needed to conserve human talent in our society.

I would now like to present another case history because it dramatizes and points up earlier failures of our society in a number of important respects. This is the story of Mr. Edwards, who was born before 1890.

*Family Background.* His mother died when he was an infant. His father died when he was nine years old. He then lived with relatives in New York City until age thirteen when he left home.

*Schooling.* He left school at age 12 with a fourth grade education and went to work. This was at the turn of the century when compulsory schooling laws were not rigidly enforced and when child labor legislation was almost unheard of.

*Work Experience, 1900–1913.* (1) Unskilled worker in wallpaper factory, four months; (2) Steam fitter's helper, plumber's helper, printer's helper, about one year; (3) Operator of drill press and punch press (learned work), about eight months in shop work; (4) Handbill distributor, house-to-house, four months; (5) Janitor in an institution, six months; (6) Tinsmith's helper, four months; (7) Itinerant worker in hotels around the country, bellhop, houseman, porter, six years; (8) Farm laborer in different parts of country, three years; and (9) Railroad car repairman's helper and bridge repairman's helper, six months.

*Accident in 1913.* While riding the rods on a freight train in 1913, he fell under the wheels, and both legs were amputated just below the knees. He was fitted with artificial limbs but never learned to use them. Upon recovery from amputation he was advised by the physician-in-charge to go into the field of selling on street corners. This vocational advice reflects 1913 attitudes toward crippled persons. The view was that industry could not use such people and that they could "earn a living" only by publicly displaying their handicap.

*Work Experience, 1913–1943.* Sold newspapers, miniature

Bibles, shoelaces, and lead pencils on street corners and was on and off of private relief and of public relief for a period of thirty years.

*Vocational Guidance Service.* Mr. Edwards came to the vocational guidance service of a city department of public relief in 1943 at the age of 55. The counselor's judgment was that this man had never made a satisfactory vocational adjustment from 1900 to 1913 nor from 1913 to 1943. The chief causes seemed to be: broken home, poor family background, limited schooling, inadequate training for the labor market, and entering labor market in the days when child labor was tolerated. Following his accident and the amputations, there were no adequate physical or vocational rehabilitation services available, and social services were also inadequate. This picture began to change, however, toward the end of the depression years. Thus, from 1941 to 1943, this man, who had married shortly after his accident and was blessed with two children, was aided by the "Lone Craftsman" organization to learn to mix paints and to paint plates at home, where it was necessary for him to stay most of the time because his wife had become bedridden with a chronic affliction. He kept house and took care of his wife, getting around with or without crutches.

*Vocational Counselor's Judgment at First Interview.* Mr. Edwards claimed he was in good physical condition with no complaints. He was quite a reader of newspapers and magazines and had followed the events of World War II with keen interest. The counselor reported that Mr. Edwards was clean of person, pleasant, cooperative, and extremely interested in the possibilities of work or of placement training. He claimed to have interests in art work, believed he could learn lettering and become a sign painter, or that he could learn machine-shop work, or that he would like to prepare for personnel work. The man appeared to have the following vocational liabilities: advanced age, crippled condition, limited schooling, poor work history, long record of dependency, and a difficult home situation. There appeared to be few, if any, vocational assets except his eagerness to become self-supporting.

*Test Results.*

1. Mr. Edwards made surprisingly high "general intelligence" test scores. In spite of the fact that his formal schooling was limited to the fourth grade which he completed at age twelve, his intelligence test scores were equal to those of the top quarter of Minnesota adults. This would be equivalent to three or four years of high school work.

2. High scores on the four Minnesota Spatial Relations Form Boards and the Minnesota Paper Form Board suggested mechanical aptitude of a high order. He ranked at the 83rd percentile and 85th percentile points of Minnesota adults on these two tests.

3. Surprisingly good scores were made on the Bell Adjustment Inventory. These probably reflect an eagerness to put his best foot forward in order to facilitate his job-planing and job-getting ambitions.

4. On the Kuder Preference Record his peak scores were 70th percentile in Mechanical, 90th percentile in Artistic, 70th percentile in Social Service, and 64th percentile in Clerical. He was, however, at the 12th percentile in Persuasive which corresponds with his "*Retiring*" score on the Bell. Both of these low scores are incompatible with the sales work he had attempted from 1913 to 1943.

*Vocational Plans.* He was enthusiastic about entering a defense plant machine-shop on-the-job training program where he would be required to work ten hours a day. He was placed in such a plant in June, 1943. The employer had already learned that physically handicapped persons with better than average mechanical ability could quickly learn to become good production workers.

*Follow-up.* Two weeks after placement, he reported he was having difficulty reading micrometers because his glasses were so scratched and in such poor repair. An eye examination and new glasses removed this difficulty.

Two months later, he reported he was working 60 hours a week and enjoying the work. His employer also reported that he was making an excellent job adjustment.

In November, he reported he was still working 60 hours a week, was well satisfied with his job but that he became exhausted before the end of the shift. He was fearful that he would not be able to keep up to the quality-of-work standards. He believed a reduction in hours per day would be helpful and was advised to consult his employer.

In the middle of December, he discussed his home situation and what could be done medically for his wife. Social Services aided at this point.

In 1946, three years after reporting to the Vocational Guidance Service, he came in voluntarily to report on his war and postwar work experiences. The record is as follows: (1) He spent one year in the defense plant which then laid off most of the workers because of defense cutbacks; (2) he then spent four months at another company but was laid off because of reduction in force; (3) he spent one year in another company but was laid off because of shortage of materials; (4) he next spent four months at another company but was laid off because of shortage of materials; and, finally, (5) he was rehired for the same job by the same company but was laid off after one month because of shortage of materials.

At this time, follow-up reports from his several employers

indicated that he had established a good work history and a good reputation as a competent worker on each job he held from 1943 through March, 1946. Furthermore, he had become a self-respecting, tax-paying citizen and at no time was in need of private or public relief. But disaster struck when he lost all of his possessions in a fire and, with unemployment compensation benefits terminated, it was necessary for Mr. Edwards to go on relief again. He is now receiving his old age pension and social security benefits and has remained out of the job market since March, 1946.

*Implications.* The case of Mr. Edwards illustrates a general failure of our society, in the past, to recognize and to utilize "better than average scholastic and mechanical aptitude" from the time he left school at the turn of the century to the time of a national emergency. It also illustrates that an occupationally maladjusted person, even though handicapped educationally, physically, occupationally, and by age for job competition, can, through appropriate vocational testing and vocational counseling, become a productive and self-respecting worker. Had adequate educational, guidance, and social service facilities been available when this man was a youngster it is probable that he might have made a far greater contribution to society throughout his life. Here, again, is a concrete example of what we mean when we stress the importance of the conservation and optimum utilization of our human resources. Manpower shortages are centering attention on this problem area with the result that we are making real headway in utilizing hitherto neglected sources of manpower.[2]

2. An excellent survey of the current situation has been reported by Dael Wolfle in *America's Resources of Specialized Talent,* Harper and Brothers, 1954.

At the present time there is widespread concern that a considerable proportion of our abler high school graduates do not go on to college. The provision of vastly increased funds for scholarships will help, but the problem is not due solely to lack of finances. There is a serious motivation problem, too, that needs attention. Early identification of the gifted and intensification of our educational and counseling efforts with such youngsters, together with the extension of our counseling programs to include the parents of the gifted, will be needed to cope with this problem of under-utilization.

The current shortage of engineers and scientists is receiving nationwide attention at the present time. Positive programs to interest more youngsters in these fields by improving instruction in mathematics and science in our high schools and by investing vast sums of money in museums of science and industry in our larger centers of population are needed and will undoubtedly be effective. But those responsible for these programs must not impose them upon youngsters who are lacking in mathematical aptitude or who have no genuine interests in science or engineering. It might also be well to point out that engineering colleges and industry must accept the challenge of optimally utilizing the scientists and engineers who are now in and will continue to enter the labor market. Perhaps we need to develop educational programs that will train increased numbers of draftsmen and scientific aids who can release many engineers and scientists from wasting their talents on routine tasks. It is with a view to facilitating this kind of attack that the University of Minnesota Industrial Relations Center has undertaken to develop specialized functional engineering vocational interest scales for Strong's Vocational Interest Blank. Dr. Wilbur Layton of our Student Counseling Bureau has constructed an effective aptitude test for freshman engineers. In addition, Dr. Marvin Dunnette has developed the Minnesota Enginering Analogies Test (1955) to aid in the selection and differential placement of engineering graduates. In brief, we would emphasize the importance of providing for and improving the vocational counseling of prospective engineers and scientists in high schools, colleges, engineering schools, graduate schools, and in industry. If these provisions are not made all along the line, it is likely that frantic efforts being made to remedy current shortages will involve a tragic maladjustment of many individuals who should have been oriented toward other occupational goals and objectives.

Other neglected sources of manpower have already been touched upon, such as those who are occupationally misclassified in the labor market. Hope for prevention of such occupational misclassification lies in the direction of improved counseling services in the schools, gearing the vocational portions of our educational programs to the real needs of business and industry, expanding the testing and counseling work in the local offices of our public employment service, and the adoption of a differential placement point of view in personnel departments in business and industry. I would like to emphasize this last point. The widespread practice of having separate employment departments in a given company for the hiring of factory workers, of clerical workers, and of salesmen is based on the false assumption that applicants for work can and do correctly classify themselves. Many applicants, however, are unaware of their own potentialities and accept whatever occupational classification may have been imposed upon them by their work histories and their prior experiences in the labor market. This merely perpetuates whatever occupational misclassifications have occurred. To overcome these serious errors, the personnel department of each company should supervise the hiring for all segments of the business and should assume responsibility for properly classifying all applicants for employment with that company. This vocational guidance point of view has only recently been hinted at in Tiffin's *Industrial Psychology* (1942) and in Robert Thorndike's book on *Personnel Selection* (1949). And, now, what I call "the Minnesota point of view" toward personnel work in business and industry is set forth in elaborate detail in the recent book by Drs. C. Harold Stone and William Kendall entitled *Effective Personnel Selection Procedures* (1956).

Another neglected source of manpower has already been hinted at earlier. I refer to the under-utilization of the physically handicapped. Systematic efforts to aid in the rehabilitation of the physically handicapped veteran and nonveteran go back to the early 1920's. The aim was worthy, but the means available were inadequate. It is a fact that rehabilitation workers, then, were almost wholly untrained. The procedure consisted primarily of asking the physically handicapped person what training he desired and then promptly providing it. If and when failure to profit from training ensued, the physically handicapped person was transferred to some other training course or school without inquiry as to whether or not it, too, was inappropriate. This process continued during the 1920's and 1930's with an appalling waste of time and money, and was accompanied by frustrated ambitions on the part of the handicapped persons and the rehabilitation workers as well. During the mid-thirties a radical shift was made in Minnesota when vocational psychologist Donald Dabelstein was put in charge of the state program. At about the same time, a demonstration of vocational counseling procedures was introduced into the Minneapolis VA Hospital. This was followed by the development of VA Guidance Centers during World War II and the development of Vocational Counseling Services in VA hospitals. But this tremendous expansion of vocational counseling services fell far short of the type and quality of services needed because of the lack of properly trained and qualified vocational counseling psychologists. This lack is now being remedied by the PhD vocational counselor training program inaugurated by the VA in 1952 and by the Federal sponsorship of a similar MA training program for vocational counselors of the physically handicapped at the state level which was begun in 1955. The net results of these two training programs will be to increase rapidly the numbers of well-trained vocational counselors of the physically handicapped. And I am proud to announce that another Minnesota trained PhD who has specialized in this area of work is author of a soon-to-be-published textbook on this subject. The author is Lloyd H. Lofquist, and the title of his book is *Vocational Counseling with the Physically Handicapped,* published in the Century Psychology Series.

May I add just a word of warning about the responsibilities of those who benefit from these improved training programs in our graduate schools? It would be a calamity if these newly trained vocational counselors should become so engrossed in theories about personality development and the counseling process itself that they failed to aid the counselee in formulating practical plans that really led to jobs and good job adjustments.

In the meantime, education of employers and of their personnel directors has been intensified to the point where resistance to the hiring of properly qualified, physically handicapped persons has been steadily reduced. There is every reason for optimism today over the prospects for a vast improvement in our utilization of the physically handicapped. Here, again, is an area in which the idea of maximum conservation of human talent is on the threshold of realization.

Another neglected source of manpower lies in our failure to utilize the ever increasing number and proportion of older persons in our society. Private pension plans force compulsory retirement of thousands who are able and willing to continue at productive work. These same plans, plus unfavorable attitudes toward the productivity of older persons, tend to set arbitrary hiring-age limits at about 40 or 45. Thanks to Dr. Lillien J. Martin, Dr. Walter R. Miles, Dr. Sidney L. Pressey, Dr. Irving Lorge, and others, the facts are now rapidly accumulating to show that age alone is a poor index of competence. Our own Industrial Relations Center has also conducted research on this problem and, more recently, has cooperated with the Public Employment Service in attempting, through research, to measure the magnitude of the problem and to study ways and means of coping with it. It is our hope that adequate age norms can be set up for the better aptitude tests now available. We also urgently need to conduct controlled experiments on the efficacy of the vocational counseling and differential placement of older persons in business and industry. Here is a major challenge that must be attacked and solved if we are to maximize the conservation of human talent among our senior citizens.

One final neglected source of manpower comprises minority groups. Because of widespread discrimination in employment, many members of many minority groups are never permitted to realize their full employment potential. Since vocational psychology must adhere to the principle of employment on the basis of merit, the vocational counselor is necessarily thrust into the midst of controversy. He will, therefore, welcome FEPC laws on the national, state, and local level. At the present writing such laws seem to be spreading at the state and local level. In Minnesota, our first FEPC law came in Minneapolis on January 1, 1947, and finally after five biennial sessions of the legislature it became state law in 1955. And other cities in our state have also adopted local ordinances setting up Fair Employment Practices Commissions. At the present time, state FEPC laws have been adopted in thirteen states, and local FEPC ordinances have been adopted in eleven communities. In addition, an increasing number of state and local Councils on Human Rights and Councils on Human Relations are paving the way for more FEPC legislation to come.

The breaking down of discrimination barriers not only serves to open up employment opportunities to qualified applicants regardless of race or creed, but it also tends to force employers to adopt more objective and scientific employment procedures. Employers must do so in order to protect themselves against unfounded charges of discrimination. This fact has accelerated the demand by employers for professionally trained personnel workers and personnel psychologists to install objective methods of hiring qualified applicants regardless of creed or color.

FEPC laws, however, are not self-enforcing. Their effectiveness, obviously, depends upon public opinion. For this reason, the vocational psychologist must aid citizens and citizen groups who are engaged in the struggle to open up and to maintain nondiscriminatory employment opportunities for everyone in our democratic society. Of course, this also means that our educational and training opportunities must likewise be provided on a nondiscriminatory basis in order that the potential abilities of every person may be identified and developed to the highest possible degree. Until this total program is fully realized in the East, the West, the North, and the South, we shall perpetuate the present inexcusable waste of precious human resources.

I have attempted to present some of the challenging problems involved in the conservation of human talent. In doing so, I have stressed the importance of vocational psychology with emphasis on the role of educational and vocational counseling in reducing and preventing occupational maladjustment in our society. Although we have made substantial progress in this regard, we are now only on the threshold of achieving some of the goals set forth so ably by the pioneers in this field. I refer, of course, to the work of Muensterberg, Thorndike, Yerkes, Terman, Scott, Hollingworth, Poffenberger, Bingham, Strong, Thurstone, Viteles,

Burt, and Toops. Fortunately, a growing number of our younger psychologists have seen the same vision and will carry on with even greater vigor and competence.

### *References*

Counts, G. S. The social status of occupations: a problem in vocational guidance. *Sch. Rev.*, 1925, 33, 16–27.

Deeg, Maethel E., & Paterson, D. G. Changes in social status of occupations. *Occupations*, 1947, 25, 205–208.

Dunnette, M. *Manual for the Minnesota Engineering Analogies Test.* New York: The Psychological Corporation, 1955.

Paterson, D. G., & Stone, C. H. Dissatisfaction with life work among adult workers. *Occupations*, 1942, *21*, 219–221.

Proctor, W. M., & Ward, Helen. Relation of general intelligence to the persistence of educational and vocational plans of high school pupils. *J. educ. Res.*, 1923, *7*, 277–288.

Roper, E. The fortune quarterly survey: XI, Part 5. *Fortune*, 1938, *17*, 86–88.

Thorndike, R. *Personnel selection.* New York: John Wiley & Sons, Inc., 1949.

Tiffin, J. *Industrial psychology.* New York: Prentice-Hall, Inc., 1942.

Stone, C. H., & Kendall, W. *Effective personnel selection procedures.* New York: Prentice-Hall, Inc., 1956.

Yoder, D., Paterson, D. G., *et al. Local labor market research.* Minneapolis: University of Minnesota Press, 1948.

*Cyril Burt*

# *The Inheritance of Mental Ability*[1]

## *The Problem of Individual Differences*

In Britain as in America, the earliest applications of the new techniques of mental testing were concerned chiefly with the lower end of the intellectual scale. They were readily accepted as practical aids to the doctor in diagnosing the mentally deficient, and to the teacher in discriminating the temporarily retarded from the irremediably dull. It was Bingham's firm belief that: "in the long run it would be even more profitable to discover and aid the bright and the supernormal than to ascertain and provide for the dull and defective."

In this country the traditional method of dealing with the problem was by means of what was popularly known as "the scholarship system." British teachers and parents were apt in those days to think of scholarships rather as a means for rewarding hard work than as a device for detecting and assisting im-

1. This paper is based on the Walter Van Dyke Bingham Memorial Lecture given at University College, London, May 21, 1957. It was first published in the *American Psychologist*, 1958, vol. 13, no.1 (January), pp. 1–15.

pecunious talent. But considerable misgiving was felt over the erratic local distribution not only of scholarship winners but also of defectives. It was indeed widely affirmed that these variations in the numbers were "largely the result of the injustice of the ordinary methods of examination." Accordingly, in 1913 the London County Council took the unprecedented step of appointing an official psychologist. His chief duties were to act as referee for what were sometimes known as "problem children"—particularly in disputed cases of feeblemindedness and of scholarship ability.

In the surveys that I carried out in this capacity I found that, in the poorer districts of the East End, there were three times as many certified defectives, eight times as many backward pupils, but only one-tenth the number of scholarship winners as were reported in the well-to-do areas of London. Who or what was to blame: the teachers, the homes, the traditional examination in arithmetic and English? Or the fact that the varying modicum of ability bestowed on each child was irretrievably fixed at birth? Environment or heredity, those seemed to be the alternative explanations; and each had its own enthusiastic advocates. As a rule the social reformers gave one answer and the psychologists the opposite.

During the nineteenth century the main champions of social reform were the philosophical radicals: Bentham, James and John Mill, and their various followers. Their motto was the maxim of Helvétius: *l'éducation peut tout;* or, as James Mill put it, "if education cannot do everything, there is hardly anything it cannot do." In psychology, their one basic law was the law of association; and the wide differences between one individual and another they attributed solely to the cumulative effects of association, through the operation of "habit, custom, training, and environmental opportunity or deprivation."

By the beginning of the twentieth century, however, most

British psychologists had abandoned this simple creed. Impressed by the novel doctrines of the evolutionary school, they began to follow Darwin, Spencer, Huxley, and Galton in holding that the laws of heredity and individual variation applied to men as well as to animals, to mind as well as to body. "It is not so much," said Karl Pearson, "that the slums create the dullards, but rather that the duller stocks gravitate automatically to the slums." It followed that the only cure would be to start breeding citizens as we bred race horses, prize rabbits, or pedigree pups. Huxley's celebrated essay on the "Natural Inequality of Man" won over the few who still wavered. Most teachers were already converted by firsthand experience under the new scheme of universal education.

However, during the last few decades psychologists have been gradually discovering that the problem is far more complicated than either side had originally assumed. And, largely as a result, there has been yet another swing of the polemical pendulum. In part this is due to a reluctance to support what G. K. Chesterton once described as "the modernized dogma of predestination—a dogma calculated to paralyse all progress towards a welfare state"; in part it has been due to a fuller appreciation of the possibilities of experience and learning, which in turn has involved a reversion to something like a rejuvenated belief in the fundamental law of association.

To the British psychologist the experimental work on "conditioning" seemed to offer a more precise interpretation, on a more adequate basis, of the traditional doctrine of association as preached by Hartley and Mill; and the behaviourist school was widely welcomed as substituting a more profitable line of practical research for inconclusive speculations about heredity and innate endowment. As a result, we find contemporary educationists reminding each other of Bagley's well known dictum that, "except for a few cases of pathological deficiency, the factor of heredity plays a very small part in human life, as compared with the factor of environment" (1912); while several of their psychological colleagues quote with approval the pronouncements of Watson: "there are inheritable differences in structure, but we no longer believe in inherited capacities." "Give me," he adds, "a dozen healthy infants, and my own world to bring them up in, and I'll guarantee to train any one of them to become any type of specialist I might select—doctor, lawyer, artist, merchant-chief, and even beggar-man or thief" (1931, p. 104).

A glance through the current literature will show that, for the most part, the hypotheses which our younger psychologists desire to challenge are the two propositions which, at the beginning of the century, were accepted almost without question as justifying the organization of our system of education: first, the hypothesis of general ability, i.e., the view that "up to adolescence the chief differences distinguishing individual pupils are differences in 'general intelligence'"—a view which led the Chief Inspector of Schools to declare that, "with a few exceptions, each pupil may be taught in the same class for every subject, or, if mentally defective, sent to a special school on the ground that he is defective all round"; secondly, the hypothesis of mental inheritance, i.e., the view that the wide differences in the degree of general ability exhibited by various pupils were due mainly to genetic endowment.

## *The Hypothesis of General Ability*

Of these two hypotheses the first was firmly rejected by the report of the "Norwood Committee"—a report which strongly influenced the reorganization of our national education as envisaged in the Education Act of 1944. The committee maintained that children differed far more in quality of ability than in amount; and recommended a tripartite classification of "secondary" schools, based on the doctrine that pupils fall into three main types: a literary or abstract type, to be educated at "grammar schools"; a mechanical or technical type, to be educated at "technical schools"; and a concrete or practical type to be educated at "modern schools." This conception was supported by several leading psychologists who argued that "the statistical analyses of Thurstone disclose no evidence for Spearman's factor of general ability, but only a number of 'primary abilities,' each more or less specialized" (Burt, 1943b).

The scheme has not worked out in actual practice so successfully as was hoped; and the proposal itself at once stimulated a large number of new inquiries. Those who still defend the tripartite theory seem to overlook the vast and varied character of the evidence that has since become available on the issue thus raised. As a rule they content themselves with citing one particular line of reasoning—usually the statistical. If, however, we take a wider view, we shall find that there are three or four independent chains of converging arguments, none perhaps irrefragable by itself, but all of them tending to rehabilitate the older view. The evidence on which these inferences rest is drawn from many different fields: introspection, observation, biology and neurology, as well as statistical research.

In point of fact, the distinction between "general ability" and "special abilities" was due, not (as is so widely supposed) to Spearman but rather to Francis Galton, from whom Spearman, as he expressly states in his earlier papers, originally borrowed it. Spearman, however, went on to deny the existence of "special abilities" which Galton had supported, on the ground that they were "just relics or revivals of the obsolete theory of faculties" (1927). It is this aspect of the Spearman doctrine that the modern educationist repudiates, and with it he is a little too ready to discard "general intelligence" as well.

However, even Galton had been partly anticipated by previous writers who, in a vague and inchoate fashion, had inculcated a somewhat similar doctrine on the basis of speculative arguments, partly introspective, partly biological. Introspection, so the faculty school had claimed, revealed a sharp distinction between intellectual or cognitive qualities on the one hand and emotional or orectic qualities on the other. Spencer and his followers accepted this distinction, and supplemented it with biological arguments, which in those days were almost equally conjectural. During the evolution of the animal kingdom, and again during the development of each individual, the fundamental capacity which Spencer termed intelligence

> . . . becomes [so he tells us] progressively differentiated into a hierarchy of more specialized cognitive capacities—sensory, perceptual, associative, and ratiocinative, much as the trunk of a growing tree ramifies into boughs and twigs (1870, Part iv).

Later writers were not so sure that the term cognition really furnished the best differentia: for them the real distinction was between directive or adaptive processes on the one hand and valuative or dynamic processes on the other; "intelligence," said Sully, "steers like a rudder; emotion and interest supply the steam." A similar reinterpretation has more recently been proposed by Piaget in his book on *The Psychology of Intelligence* (1950, pp. 4ff.).

Far more convincing to my mind is the neurological evidence. The alternative doctrine of distinct and independent abilities drew much of its support from early experiments on cerebral localization. These, it was claimed,

> . . . appear to indicate that distinct functions—motor, sensory, perceptual, associative, linguistic, and the like—can be assigned to distinct and definite centres or areas within the brain.

And this conclusion was apparently corroborated by the maps of cell structure subsequently produced by histologists like Campbell, Brodmann, and von Economo. Their inferences, however, have been severely criticized by more recent workers, like Bok, Lorente de Nò, and, at University College, by D. A. Sholl (1956). Few of the older map makers (he says) realized "the enormous amount of variability that exists between individual human brains." In their studies of comparable cortical areas from different specimens of *Ateles* Lashley and Clark have shown that the differences between different individuals are at least as large as the differences upon which the distinction of "architectonic areas" was based (1946). Hence it now seems clear that the charts that used to figure in popular textbooks "greatly exaggerated the amount and the definiteness of the alleged localization, both as regards structure and as regards function."

After all, as Sherrington so frequently pointed out, in any one individual each anatomical tissue—skin, bone, hair, or muscle—tends to be of the same general character all over the body: minor local variations are often discernible; but in the same individual the variations are much slighter than those between one individual and another; and we should naturally expect the same to hold good of nerve tissue. Bolton's studies of the cerebral cortex, both in normal and defective persons, suggest that the quality of the nervous tissue in any given individual tends to be predominantly the same throughout: in low-grade defectives, for example, the nerve cells tend to be "visibly deficient in number, in branching, and in regularity of arrangement in every part of the cortex." The clinical work of Hughlings Jackson, the experimental researches of Sherrington, and the microscopical studies of the infant brain carried out more recently by Conel and de Crinis, seem in many ways to provide increasing confirmation for Spencer's theory of a "hierarchy of neural functions," developing stage by stage out of a simpler basic activity into higher and more specialized forms. Even if we cannot wholly accept Lashley's doctrine of the "mass action" of the brain, nevertheless the actual facts that he has reported are far more in keeping with a theory of general ability (and minor special abilities) than with a theory of major "special abilities" and no general factor. And Sholl himself concludes that "intelligence," like retentivity, is a "general attribute of all cortical tissue" (1956, p. 111).

Each of the foregoing arguments—from introspection, from biology, and from neurology—is admittedly inconclusive. The most we could so far claim is that, when taken in combination, the evidence from each of these separate fields sets up a fairly strong a priori probability in favour of Galton's twofold theory of general abilities plus special. It is at this point, therefore, that the psychologist is tempted to invoke the aid of statistical analysis. In my view, the function of statistics, at any rate in psychological research, is simply to provide a more rigorous method of testing alternative hypotheses. How then do the various hypotheses that confront us stand up to this ordeal?

Each of the three main suggestions leads to distinctive corollaries which are open to statistical verification. First of all, if, as Thorndike held, there was no such thing as a general factor, but only a set of independent abilities, then the cross-correlation between the tests or assessments for those abilities should be zero, or at least nonsignificant. They are not: they are always both significant and positive. Secondly, if, as Spearman maintained, there were no such thing as special abilities but only a single general factor, the intercorrelations for every test should diminish proportionately in the same descending order (except, of course, for nonsignificant deviations due to sampling and the like): in technical language, the table of intercorrelations should constitute a matrix of rank one. It does not.

The third hypothesis assumes the presence of both general and special abilities. In the early article (1909) to which I have already referred,[2] I endeavoured to apply to the correlations between mental tests the procedure which Karl Pearson had already elaborated for use with measurements of bodily characteristics. In this way I sought to compare each of my various tables of observed coefficients with the best fitting set of theoretical values deduced from the hypothesis of a single "general ability" only; this hypothetical ability was redefined as the "highest common factor" entering into all the processes measured in any given table.[3] The fit was moderately good, but by no means perfect. The differences between the observed and the theoretical values were accordingly tested for statistical significance; and the result was to disclose small but significant clusters of residual correlations, common to certain limited groups of tests

2. Those to whom this earlier (1909) paper is inaccessible will find the essential figures from one of the tables reproduced in books by Freeman (1926) and Thorndike (1914); Garnett (1921) reprints not only the observed values, but, beneath them, the theoretical values, the discrepancies, and the probable errors, as I myself had done. It should be noted that the procedure subsequently developed by Spearman (1927) was rather different. He preferred to secure independent assessments for intelligence, based on teachers' ratings, examination results, or, in later inquiries, the results of one or two accredited tests, and use them as "reference values." In other words, he used an *external* criterion; whereas I have used an *internal* criterion or "factor" derived from the intercorrelations themselves. My reasons were that both examination results and teachers' assessments were commonly influenced by the child's capacity to learn, i.e., by his memory, rather than by his sheer intelligence, and thus often reflected what the child had actually acquired rather than his innate capacity.

3. The simplified formula used for this purpose in most of these earlier researches (1917, p. 53) was the same as that subsequently adopted by Thurstone under the name of the centroid formula (1935, p. 94, Equation 13). When in addition "special abilities" were studied as well as "general ability," they were regarded as "group factors" obtainable by an arithmetical rotation of the "bipolar" factor matrix. I may add that we encountered a certain amount of evidence indicating that several of these special abilities were also largely dependent on heredity, but space does not permit me to deal with them here.

only, thus plainly indicating the presence of certain supplementary abilities. This seemed definitely to clinch the double hypothesis put forward by Galton. Precisely the same conclusion was reached in many later analyses carried out both by myself and by other workers with larger numbers of pupils and a greater variety of tests (Burt, 1914–1931, 1917).

The factorization of correlations between persons and between successive occasions (with the same persons and tests) revealed, or at least very plainly confirmed, the constant presence of a random factor, which appeared to be due, not merely to sampling as ordinarily understood, but to something essentially characteristic of the working of the mind or brain. A somewhat similar conclusion has been independently reached by neurologists like Beurle, Cragg and Temperley, and Uttley and Sholl. Thus the type of "neuronal connectivity" suggested by the histological study of dendritic fibres strongly suggests "the semi-random arrangement of a machine working largely in accordance with the principles of probability" (Sholl, 1956).[4] This partly

4. This is not the same as the "sampling theory" of Thomson, which maintains that the apparent emergence of "factors" is "a result of the laws of chance and not of any psychological laws": like all simplified theories, it seems to amplify just one aspect of mental process, at the expense of denying all the rest. What is needed is a model which will combine the "integrative action" of the nervous system with its "stochastic action." As I have suggested elsewhere (*Psychometrika,* 3, p. 160), the mathematical model which most effectively does this is a classificatory model derived from Pearson's method of principal axes. The mechanical model would resemble, not the homeostat of Ashby or the mechanical tortoise of Grey Walter, but rather a classification machine like that proposed by Uttley and Sholl. Similarly a stochastical induction machine would seem to reproduce the results of human learning far better than the model adopted by Hull and his followers. It is therefore tempting to suggest that what has been called the A/S ratio—i.e., the proportionate amount of "association cortex" with which either a species or an organism is endowed at birth—would form an index primarily of the amount of its intelligence and only incidentally of its capacity to learn.

agrees with, though it is by no means identical with, the doctrine of "equipotentiality" put forward by Lashley; and thus further supports the value of factorial procedures as a means of investigating variations in mental ability.

However, what is far more important from the practical standpoint of educational guidance is this: in nearly every factorial study of cognitive ability, the general factor commonly accounts for quite 50% of the variance (rather more in the case of the young child, rather less with older age groups) while each of the minor factors accounts for only 10% or less. With increasing age, the "group factors," which represent special abilities, contribute increasing amounts to the total variance; and this fact lends further support to the view that, as a result of maturation, cognitive ability progressively differentiates and tends to become more and more specialized (Burt, 1954).

Be that as it may, whatever be our views on the various biological or neurological issues, we may, I think, safely say this: for purposes of prediction—forecasting what this or that individual child is likely to do in school or in after-life—the general factor is by far the most important, though admittedly not our only, guide. For all practical purposes, almost every psychologist—even former opponents of the concept of general intelligence, like Thorndike, Brown, Thomson, and Thurstone—seems in the end to have come round to much the same conclusion, even though, for theoretical purposes, each tends to reword it in a modified terminology of his own. And thus today, save for one or two occasional attacks, current psychological criticism is not so much concerned with the problem of "general intelligence," but is directed rather against the second of our two initial propositions: the assumption, namely, that individual differences in intelligence are hereditary or innate.

### *The Genetic Component*

Here three distinct questions seem to be involved: (*a*) what evidence is there for the *fact* of inheritance, (*b*) what precisely is the *mode* in which intelligence is inherited, and (*c*) what is the *relative importance* of the genetic factor as compared with the environmental?

*The Fact.* In controversies about the facts of mental heredity most critics have tended to assume that the two causal agencies commonly discussed—heredity and environment—are not merely antithetical but mutually exclusive. The environmentalists apparently suppose that, once they have shown that intelligence tests are affected by environment, it follows that all differences in intelligence are due to nothing but environment. Similarly the thoroughgoing hereditarian is apt to talk as though he believed that differences in intelligence were due to nothing but genetic constitution. This is the old familiar fallacy which I am tempted to label "nothing-buttery." In point of fact, with a few rare exceptions, like eye colour or serological differences in the blood, every observable characteristic that geneticists have studied has proved to be the product of the joint action of both heredity and environment. There are, in short, no such things as hereditary characters: there are only hereditary tendencies.

Now, where two contributory factors, such as heredity and environment, are likely to be involved, the obvious procedure will be to keep first one and then the other as constant as possible, and observe the results in either case.

1. *Uniform environment.* As psychological consultant to the London County Council, I had free access to orphanages and other residential institutions, and to the private files of case records giving the history of the various inmates. My co-workers and I were thus able to study large numbers of children who had been transferred thither during the earliest weeks of infancy, and

had been brought up in an environment that was much the same for all. To our surprise we found that individual differences in intelligence, so far from being diminished, varied over an unusually wide range. In the majority of cases, they appeared to be correlated with differences in the intelligence of one or both of the parents. Some of the most striking instances were those of illegitimate children of high ability: often the father (so the case records showed) had been a casual acquaintance, of a social and intellectual status well above that of the mother, and had taken no further interest in the child. In such cases it is out of the question to attribute the high intelligence of the child to the special cultural opportunities furnished by the home environment, since his only home has been the institution.[5]

2. *Uniform heredity.* To secure cases in which the children's genetic endowment is the same, we may turn to assessments obtained from monozygotic or "identical" twins. The mother is not infrequently unable or unwilling to bring up two children at the same time, and one twin is consequently sent to a relative or to a foster home. Owing to the strong popular prejudice against separating twins, she not unnaturally tries, as a rule, to keep these arrangements secret. But patient and tactful inquiries show that cases of twins brought up in different environments almost from birth are in fact much commoner than is usually believed. We have now collected over 30 such cases (1943c, 1955). I re-

5. Details are given in the various *Annual Reports of the Psychologist to the London County Council* (Burt, 1914–1931) and are summarized in Burt, 1943c. In the recent symposium on *Quantitative Inheritance* (1952), Woolf, quoting a later paper of mine, regrets that I have "based such far reaching conclusions on the study by Barbara Burks . . . covering only 214 foster children" (1928). But the principal basis for my own conclusion was a series of investigations in residential schools under the LCC covering in the course of years over 600 cases. I cited Burks' inquiry merely to show how an independent investigator in a different country had arrived at much the same figures as my own.

produce the more important correlations for the twins in Table 1 and have added for comparison corresponding coefficients obtained from other pairs, both related and unrelated. As regards intelligence the outstanding feature is the high correlation between the final assessments for the monozygotic twins, even when reared apart: it is almost as high as the correlation between two successive testings for the same individuals. On the other hand, with school attainments the correlations are much lower for twins reared separately than for twins reared together in the same home.

Several of our critics—Heim and Maddox, for example—have cited the account of analogous cases (described by Newman and others) as proving that intelligence is dependent on environment. Thus, to take an oft-quoted pair, "Helen," who had been trained as a teacher, scored with the Stanford-Binet tests an IQ of 116; whereas her twin sister, "Gladys," brought up for much of her childhood in an isolated district of the Canadian Rockies, scored only 92. But, says Newman, her score

> . . . was higher than we might expect considering her scant education; and . . . it seems certain that the great deficiency in education had inhibited the development of the rather high grade of mental ability with which she was *endowed by heredity* (1942, pp. 136–144).

Thus Newman's interpretation in no way conflicts with ours.

It is sometimes alleged (Maddox, 1957) that, since twins are born at the same time, the intrauterine environment must have been the same for both before birth, even if later on their environments differ widely, and that quite conceivably it is the former that is crucial. As it happens, however, this rather gratuitous assumption reverses the actual facts. Embryological and obstetric records show that, particularly with twins developed from split ova, the position of each in the uterus, and the subse-

Table 1. Correlations between mental and scholastic assessments.

| | Identical twins reared together | Identical twins reared apart | Nonidentical twins reared together | Siblings reared together | Siblings reared apart | Unrelated children reared together |
|---|---|---|---|---|---|---|
| Mental | | | | | | |
| "Intelligence" | | | | | | |
| Group Test | .944 | .771 | .542 | .515 | .441 | .281 |
| Individual Test | .921 | .843 | .526 | .491 | .463 | .252 |
| Final Assessment | .925 | .876 | .551 | .538 | .517 | .269 |
| Scholastic | | | | | | |
| General Attainments | .898 | .681 | .831 | .814 | .526 | .535 |
| Reading and Spelling | .944 | .647 | .915 | .853 | .490 | .548 |
| Arithmetic | .862 | .723 | .748 | .769 | .563 | .476 |

quent development, is liable to differ widely (Burt and Howard, 1956, pp. 123ff. and refs.).

I think, therefore, that it may be safely said that, apart from the influence of some preconceived theory, few psychologists nowadays would be inclined to contest the mere fact of mental inheritance: the most that can be plausibly alleged is that its influence is comparatively slight and distinctly elusive.

*The Mode of Inheritance.* The majority of those who still question the importance of mental inheritance, and many of those who support it, seem by preference to adopt entirely antiquated notions of the way in which inheritable characteristics are transmitted. If, as I have maintained, mental capacities are dependent on the physical characteristics of the brain (or, to speak a little more precisely, on the structural and biochemical qualities of the nervous system), then we should expect those capacities to be inherited in accordance with the same principles that govern the inheritance of physical characteristics; and these principles (except for obscure and apparently exceptional instances of extranuclear heredity) are essentially those commonly associated with the name of Mendel. Many British psychologists, however, feel a strong and not unreasonable prejudice against applying "atomistic theories like Mendel's" to explain the facts of mental life, and consequently, so far as they admit the possibility of mental inheritance at all, still cling to the old Darwinian principle of blended inheritance. On this view heredity means "the tendency of like to beget like" (the definition quoted by one of them from the *Oxford English Dictionary*). As a result, they commonly assume that the arguments for inheritance must consist in demonstrating resemblances between the parent and his children by means of correlations. When the two parents differ, then the child is still expected to consist in an intermediate blend of both.

The approach of the modern geneticist is the reverse of all

this. As he views it, the real problem is rather to explain why in so many instances "like begets unlike." Both for the environmentalist and for the believer in blended inheritance, one of the most puzzling phenomena is the appearance, not merely of extremely dull children in the families of the well-to-do professional classes, but also of extremely bright children in families where both the cultural and the economic conditions of the parents would, one might imagine, condemn every child to hopeless failure. With the Mendelian hypothesis these anomalies are just what we should anticipate. However, the few critics who are familiar with the Mendelian explanation appear, as a rule, to suppose that it can apply only to discontinuous variations; and point out that intelligence, like stature, exhibits not discontinuous but continuous or graded variation. Hence, so they contend (sometimes citing the experiments of De Vries on "pure lines"), the apparent differences in intelligence between one individual and another must be due almost entirely to differences in environmental conditions.

Mendel himself was the first to indicate how his theory could be extended to account for this particular difficulty. When supplementing his experiments on the hybridization of peas by hybridizing beans, and (as before) crossing white flowered plants with purple, he found, that, whereas with peas the two types always sorted out with no hint of any intermediate color, with beans the offspring displayed "a whole range of hues from white to deep purple." This, he suggested, might be explained by postulating that with beans the color was determined, not by a single pair of alternative factors, but by a *number* of such pairs, each positive factor, when present, contributing a small additional amount of color. And if, as before, the recombinations are the effects of chance unions, then the resulting frequencies would obviously approximate to those of the normal curve.

However, in our early surveys of London children (1914–1931, 1917), we found that, when complete age groups were tested, the distribution of intelligence departed significantly from that of a perfect normal curve: there was a swollen tail at the lower end, due to an excess of mental defectives, and a smaller enlargement at the upper end. This and other considerations led me to put forward the tentative hypothesis that innate variations in intelligence are due partly to unifactor and partly to multifactor inheritance: i.e., they result from Mendelian factors of two main kinds (no doubt overlapping), viz., (*a*) major genes responsible for comparatively *large* deviations, usually of an abnormal type, and (*b*) multiple genes whose effects are *small, similar,* and *cumulative.*

Karl Pearson (1904) endeavoured to test the Mendelian theory in its multifactorial form by comparing its implications with actual figures obtained for height, arm length, and similar physical measurements, collected by himself and Alice Lee, from over 2,000 students and their relatives. The expected correlations which he deduced for various degrees of kinship were in every case far smaller than the observed coefficients. He therefore emphatically rejected the hypothesis of Mendelian inheritance, and fell back on the older theory of blending. However, in deriving his formulae and his expected values, Pearson relied on an oversimplified model. Contrary to what we now know to be the case, he assumed that the effect of assortative mating—the tendency of like to marry like—could be ignored as negligible, and that dominance would in every case be perfect. Ronald Fisher has since undertaken the rather formidable task of deducing more appropriate formulae, which allow for these and other complicating factors (1918). And with these refinements the calculated correlations fit Pearson's own figures as well as could be wished.

My colleagues and I have applied Fisher's methods (suitably modified) to assessments for intelligence (Burt and Howard, 1956). The data were secured in the course of surveys of the entire school population in a representative London borough, and covered nearly 1,000 pairs of siblings, together with ratings for parents, and (so far as they were accessible) grandparents, uncles and aunts, and first cousins. The final assessments for the children were obtained by submitting the marks from the group tests to the judgment of the teachers who knew the children best: where the teacher disagreed with the verdict of the marks, the child was interviewed personally, and subjected to further tests, often on several successive occasions. The assessments for the adult members of the family were naturally far less accurate. Nevertheless, in almost every case the correlations computed from the actual data agreed with the theoretical values deduced from the multifactorial hypothesis far better than with the values deduced from any other hypothesis hitherto put forward. The only appreciable discrepancy occurred in the case of first cousins. Here, as for stature, the observed correlation for intelligence is larger than the theoretical; but the difference is not statistically significant, and could readily be explained if (as has been suggested above) variations in intelligence are affected by a few major genes as well as by numerous minor genes. I may add that on sorting out figures for cousins of maternal, paternal, and mixed kinship there is also some slight evidence suggestive of sex linkage.

*The Relative Influence of Heredity and Environment.* In practical work, however, the question most frequently raised is, not whether differences in intelligence are inherited, nor even how they are inherited, but rather what is the relative influence of heredity as compared with environment. To an omnibus inquiry like this there can be no single answer. We can only try to determine, for this or that type of environment, for this or that population, and for this or that type of assessment, how far the observable results appear to be influenced by each of the two main groups of factors.

As Fisher's analysis has shown, formulae analogous to those used to deduce the expected correlations from the theoretical variances can also be devised for deducing the amount of the constituent variances from the observed correlations. I have ventured to amplify Fisher's methods (mainly on the lines of later work by Mather and Sewall Wright) so as to allow for unreliability and for the systematic effects of environment, i.e., of environmental influences which are correlated with those of heredity, as well as for random effects. The genetic contribution may be regarded as comprising two distinguishable portions: that due to the "fixable" component (or, as Fisher expresses it, to the "essential genotypes") and that due to the "nonfixable" (i.e., deviations due to dominance and similar influences). The data analysed consist of (*a*) the marks obtained from intelligence tests of the ordinary type taken just as they stand and (*b*) adjusted assessments obtained by the supplementary methods already described (Burt and Howard, 1956).

From Table 2 it will be seen that, with the crude test results, taken just as they stand, nearly 23% of the total variance appears due to nongenetic influences, i.e., to environment or to unreliability, and about 77% to genetic factors; with the adjusted assessments only about 12% (or slightly more) is apparently due to nongenetic influences and 88% to genetic factors. This of course means that the common practice of relying on tests alone —usually a group test applied once only—is by no means a satisfactory method of assessing a child's innate ability. Better assessments are obtained by submitting the test scores to the teachers for criticism or correction, and where necessary adjust-

Table 2. Analysis of variance for assessments of intelligence.

| Source | Unadjusted test scores | Adjusted assessments |
|---|---|---|
| Genetic component: | | |
| fixable | 40.51 | 47.92 |
| nonfixable | 16.65 | 21.73 |
| Assortative mating | 19.90 | 17.91 |
| Environment: | | |
| systematic | 10.60 | 1.43 |
| random | 5.91 | 5.77 |
| Unreliability | 6.43 | 5.24 |
| Total | 100.00 | 100.00 |

ing them by the methods described above. But such intensive inquiries would be too costly for routine use except in borderline cases.

Environment appears to influence the test results chiefly in three ways: (*a*) the cultural amenities of the home and the educational opportunities provided by the school can undoubtedly affect a child's performance in intelligence tests of the ordinary type, since so often they demand an acquired facility with abstract and verbal modes of expression; (*b*) quite apart from what the child may learn, the constant presence of an intellectual background may stimulate (or seem to stimulate) his latent powers by inculcating a keener motivation, a stronger interest in intellectual things, and a habit of accurate, speedy, and diligent work; (*c*) in a few rare cases illness or malnutrition during the prenatal or early postnatal stages may, almost from the very start, permanently impair the development of the child's central nervous system. The adjusted assessments may do much towards eliminating the irrelevant effects of the first two conditions; but it is doubtful whether they can adequately allow for the last.

***Limitations Involved in These Conclusions***

As in almost all scientific investigations, the hypothetical model which has formed the basis of our inquiry involves of necessity certain minor simplifications. In particular we have assumed, for purposes of calculation, a sharp distinction between the "major genes" of unifactor inheritance and the "polygenes" of multifactor inheritance, and have treated the latter as contributing equal and additive doses to the sum total of each child's innate intelligence. We have then supposed that the effects of the former would on the whole be excluded if the few obviously pathological cases (mostly found in special schools or institutions) were omitted from our final calculations. However, these assumptions have led several critics to accuse us of

> . . . disrupting the individual personality into atomic bits and discrete pieces which have subsequently to be joined together like a mosaic. . . . Personality [it is argued] is not a mosaic but a seamless whole, and hence the entire Mendelian hypothesis with its particulate genes, each producing a unit-character or adding another unit to the same character, is quite inapplicable to the facts of conscious behavior, and therefore to the study of mental capacity.

Objections of this kind could of course be used just as well to prove that a neuronic theory of the central nervous system is incompatible with the facts of conscious behaviour or of individual variations in ability, since nerve cells or "neural bonds" are equally "particulate." Nevertheless, even those neurologists who prefer to start from a "field theory" do not wholly reject the neuronic hypothesis (cf. Sholl, 1956). In both cases the difficulties raised owe their force chiefly to the fact that there is a vast series of elusive processes intervening between theory and observable results which the critic is exceedingly apt to forget.

Moreover, criticisms like those just cited plainly rest on an obsolete version of the Mendelian doctrine. No geneticist today, I imagine, accepts the hypothesis of the autonomous corpuscular gene; and the genotypic endowment of the individual can only affect the phenotypic resultant through the mediation of innumerable obscure biochemical steps.

In our original papers Howard and I tried carefully to guard against recurrent objections of this type. As we pointed out, the phrase "multiple factors" may be used to cover either (*a*) relatively numerous loci each with only two allelomorphs or (*b*) a single locus (or relatively few loci) each with numerous allelomorphs, or possibly (*c*) some combination of the two. Hypothesis *b* by itself would hardly seem to fit the facts. We are inclined to think that factors of all the various types may be operative in varying degrees, and that the attempt to classify factors or genes should not be too severely pressed.

We further assumed that in all probability the influence of such factors on the individual's observable intelligence was mainly the indirect result of their influence on the development of his central nervous system, and was presumably effected by modifying growth rates. And we expressly stated that the ultimate influence of any one "gene" upon intelligence might be but one of its multifarious consequences, and possibly a comparatively remote consequence at that. Some genes may have a larger share in the final result; others a smaller; and the rough classification of genes into "major" genes and "minor" was adopted primarily with a view to simplifying our general discussion.[6] We

6. If Mather's view that "the major genes occur only in euchromatin, while heterochromatin contains only polygenes" (Darlington and Mather, 1949, p. 151) is eventually confirmed there would be more adequate grounds for retaining a sharp distinction between the two modes of inheritance. However, this view is not universally accepted. For an alternative interpretation of the experimental results on which Mather largely relies, see the papers by Reeve and Robertson quoted in our article (Burt

ourselves find the "theory of chromosomal hierarchy," advanced by Goldschmidt (1955), especially attractive as a basis for the ultimate hierarchical differentiation of mental ability.

However, this is not the place to enlarge on these speculative interpretations. We fully admit that the simplifications involved in our hypothetical model mean that the figures finally deduced can be no more than approximations. But we maintain that the error of approximation, however large, will nevertheless be smaller than the amount of "unreliability" inevitably involved in all such measurements.

In any case we must repeat that the conclusions reached are at best only valid in reference to the particular conditions under which they were obtained. They would not necessarily hold good (*a*) of other mental traits, (*b*) of different methods of assessment, (*c*) of a population of a different genetic composition, or (*d*) of a population at a different cultural level: much less would they hold good if there were any subsequent change (*e*) in the present distribution of environmental and genetic characteristics, or (*f*) in the influences affecting their mutual interaction.[7]

### *The Inheritance of Other Mental Qualities*

The mental trait in which we have been chiefly interested is the general factor of "intelligence." This, we readily concede, is but one psychological ingredient in ordinary everyday behaviour. Our critics are accustomed to reproach us for apparently ignoring the rest. There are several obvious reasons why we have dealt

---

and Howard, 1956, p. 116). These writers incline more to what in the text I have called hypothesis *b*. But, as Howard and I contended, their alternative interpretation would affect only the method, not the results, of our statistical deductions.

7. A more detailed reply to the criticisms urged by Woolf, Heim, and Maddox appears in the issue of the *Brit. J. statist. Psychol.*, 1954, Part i.

less fully with other determinants. The first and the most conclusive is that comparatively little evidence is as yet available in regard to the genetic composition of other mental factors. We have, however, in the course of our surveys, met with an appreciable number of cases which strongly suggest the inheritability of certain specific abilities and disabilities, or rather of certain ill-defined tendencies that presumably underlie such disabilities —particularly in our studies of memory, of visual, auditory, and kinaesthetic imagery, and of verbal, numerical, artistic, and musical aptitudes (Burt, 1914–1931). We have encountered other cases which suggest the inheritability of general emotional instability, of temperamental qualities like introversion and extraversion, and of certain quasi-instinctive tendencies like sex and bad temper (or "pugnacity," as McDougall would have termed it). But emotional tendencies are always much more liable to be influenced and altered by postnatal experiences, and in any case undergo considerable changes during the developmental stages, so that all attempts at assessment are apt to be precarious. The most convincing evidence is afforded by the family histories of children brought up in orphanages or residential institutions (Burt, 1941, especially p. 14). In all these instances the evidence, such as it is, appears to indicate that each of the characteristics mentioned, cognitive and temperamental alike, is influenced both by unifactor and by multifactor modes of inheritance—the latter tending on the whole to predominate, but in varying degrees. This after all is what is commonly found in investigations on physical characteristics. Characteristics depending mainly (though not entirely) on the development of the long bones—such as arm length, leg length, stature, and perhaps the longer dimensions of the face and head—yield correlations of much the same magnitude as those obtained for general intelligence. Others, like cephalic index, breadth at hips, and particularly facial characteristics, seem to be rather more subject to the influence of single (or relatively few) genes, which often appear to exhibit almost perfect dominance. Variations in the cartilaginous features, and particularly those depending on flesh and fat, are far more readily affected by environmental influences (for data, see Tanner, 1953).

But secondly there is a practical reason for concentrating attention first of all, and chiefly, on the inheritability of general intelligence. General intelligence, as we have seen, accounts for four times as much of the variance as any other identifiable factor. Galton's pronouncement is thus fully borne out by our own results:

> . . . general ability appears far more important than special gifts; and, where the allowance granted by nature is inadequate, the keenest will and the stoutest industry must strive in vain.

Moreover, the child's innate endowment of intelligence sets an upper limit to the best he can possibly attain. No one would expect a Mongolian imbecile, with the most skilful coaching in the world, to achieve the scholastic knowledge of an average child. In the same way, no should expect a child who is innately dull to gain a scholarship to a grammar school, or one whose inborn ability is merely average to win first class honors at Oxford or Cambridge. No doubt, in any individual case the ascertainment of this upper limit can never be a matter of absolute certainty: an IQ derived from tests alone falls far short of a trustworthy indication. Hence education authorities, like life insurance companies, have to follow Butler's maxim, and take probability for their guide. They cannot, however, afford to risk a lavish expenditure on cases where there are fairly heavy odds against success.

Nevertheless, it must be owned that, in Britain at any rate, the existing administrative machinery is far less efficient than it might be. In an inquiry made just before the introduction of the Education Act of 1944 we found that "approximately 40 percent of those whose innate abilities are of university standard are failing to reach the university" (Burt, 1943c). The new arrangements proposed by the act, and the postwar changes in the economic circumstances of the various social classes, have appreciably altered the entries to "grammar schools"; but it is too early to say how far they have affected the composition of the universities. For grammar schools the entries vary considerably from one area to another and even from year to year. The general aim is apparently to provide a grammar school education for the brightest 20% of each age group; this corresponds to a border line of about 113 IQ. On this basis the round figures in Table 3 represent estimates deduced from the information so far available.

A more intensive survey of two contrasted areas ("industrial" and "prosperous") has just been published by J. E. Floud and her colleagues. Briefly their conclusion is that, in both areas, gross material handicaps have been greatly lessened, though not entirely eliminated. Nevertheless, in their view, the "problem of social wastage" is by no means overcome. The fact that, even today, a large proportion of the children from the working classes fail to reach the higher levels of scholastic instruction Floud her-

Table 3. Estimates for grammar school entries.

| | General population[a] | Proportions over +0.85 SD | Expected entries | Actual entries |
|---|---|---|---|---|
| Middle Class | 20% | .40 | .08 (40%) | 55% |
| Manual Class | 80% | .15 | .12 (60%) | 45% |
| Total | 100% | | .20 (100%) | 100% |

[a] The *Census of Great Britain* (1951) gives an estimate of 81.7 for males over 15, occupied or retired, falling into the classes of "Skilled," "Mixed," and "Unskilled" workers; these I have pooled in a single broad group.

self attributes to the way in which the "educational ladder" is still widely regarded as a "middle class prerogative," to be anxiously watched and jealously preserved (1956).

I myself should be inclined to look rather to a difference in the aims and aspirations which are traditional in the different classes. The consequences seemed clearly revealed by the differences in the after-careers of LCC scholarship winners from the lower and the middle classes respectively whom my colleagues and I have been able to follow up (cf. 1914–1931, Burt and Howard, 1956).[8] The figures show that the abler children from the working classes, even when they have obtained free places or scholarships at secondary schools of the "grammar" type, frequently fail to stay the course: by the time they are sixteen the attractions of high wages and of cheap entertainment during leisure hours prove stronger than their desire for further knowledge and skill, and easily overcome their original resolve to face a long prospect of hard sedentary work *in statu pupillari.* As a headmaster of a secondary school which receives both types of boy has put it:

---

8. Additional evidence is furnished by the report of the Central Advisory Council for Education (England) on *Early Leaving.* In 1953, at the age of entry to the grammar school (11 plus), 66% of the top intelligence group were the children of manual workers; at the end of the grammar school period the proportion had fallen to 47%. Of those who drop out, some are "premature leavers," i.e., they leave voluntarily, as soon as they are legally able to do so; others fail to reach the top form and so leave at 16: of these many even fail to secure a school leaving certificate. In such cases, the award of a special place in the grammar school would seem itself to have been a wasted effort. Nevertheless, in the long run there may be certain compensating advantages to the community as a whole: even the early leavers may have gained something from the higher education to which they have been for a while subjected, and it would surely be a misfortune were all the brightest youngsters to forsake the social class into which they were born. Their continued presence there must help, not only to elevate its tone, but also (a point too often overlooked) to prevent its genetic constitution from being wholly depleted of its better elements.

> The working class parent wants his boy to be "selected" chiefly to prove that "his child is a good as anybody else's"; having done so, he will withdraw him at the earliest possible opportunity: I do not press them, for the presence of those whose chief interest in life is television, Hollywood films, football pools, "the dogs," and "the girls" has not improved the tone of my school. And too often these "ignobler attitudes and crude ambitions" are shared by, and encouraged by, both parents and friends.

On the other hand, if I may quote the report of an experienced university teacher:

> That section of the middle class which seeks, by paying fees that it can ill afford, to assist its children to climb, *via* a "public school" or an independent "grammar school," to a University education and a good honours degree in the humaner subjects, is animated by a traditional morale which is comparatively rare in children and parents from the other classes: those who nowadays come here on grants, at no cost to themselves or their parents, are, on the whole, most irregular attendants, and the least satisfactory students.

Or, to quote a still more recent pronouncement of the High Master of St. Paul's:[9]

> The parents are themselves imbued with four traditional ideals which they hand on to their posterity: self-discipline, a community spirit, the Christian religion, and a readiness to accept social responsibility even at the sacrifice of material enjoyments—a genuine *noblesse oblige.*

Underlying all these differences in outlook I myself am tempted to suspect an innate and transmissible difference in

9. A. N. Gilkes, *Independence in Education,* 1957.

temperamental stability and in character, or in the neurophysiological basis on which such temperamental and moral differences tend to be built up. Tradition may explain much: it can hardly account for all. However, it would be idle to pursue such speculations here in the absence of more adequate data.[10]

## *Need For Further Research*

To my mind the most pressing need at the moment is for more extensive research. Hitherto the most active investigators have been research-students, with little or no experience of the ways of children or the conditions of the classroom. For the requisite

10. Since my lecture was written and delivered, some further information has become available in the data published by the Association of Universities of the British Commonwealth (*Report of an Inquiry into Applications for Admissions to Universities,* 1957). It appears that at Oxford and Cambridge only 12% of the men and 7% of the women had fathers in manual occupations; at other universities the proportions were somewhat higher, namely, 31% and 19%, respectively. Among the general population 72% of the population would fall into the manual category. The report points out that to a large extent the decline must occur during the school period, and the real reason, it is suggested, is more often lack of zeal than lack of the requisite ability. "Differing environmental influences and aspirations seem mainly responsible for the fall from 66% at the point of entry to the non-fee-paying grammar school and 36% at the point of university entry. . . . Discrimination against those of humble social origin can be virtually ruled out."

Most education authorities nowadays tend to use what are misleadingly termed "intelligence tests" as tests of suitability for a grammar school. (Such tests, as I have argued elsewhere, should rather be termed "tests of scholastic aptitude.") The original intention was that the "intelligence test" should, so far as possible, assess innate ability. Bright children with special verbal or literary abilities and interests were then to be allocated to grammar schools; and those with practical or mechanical abilities or interests, to technical schools. But for the majority the age of 11 plus is too early to make a satisfactory distinction. Hence the brightest still seem likely to be sent to secondary schools of the grammar type rather than to a technical school, even if more suited to the latter.

facilities, and for any supplementary information they may want, they have to rely on the goodwill of the busy teacher. And one important factor is still more often overlooked: the motivation of the children themselves. This takes two obvious forms. There is first what may be called direct or short distance motivation. As actual trial has repeatedly shown, neither pupils nor students are likely to exert their full powers in a test conducted merely in the interests of someone else's research; but when the examinees' entrance to a grammar school or university depends on their performances, the average score may rise 5 to 10 IQ points higher. Secondly, there are the effects of indirect or long distance motivation: the influence of parental attitudes, of teachers' exhortations, and (most of all perhaps with British lads) of the social pressure that arises from the opinions and the comments of their school fellows, and from the tone and atmosphere of the school or class to which the pupil belongs. It is therefore hardly surprising if the results obtained in mere academic researches are at times disappointing, and evince a comparatively low reliability.

I myself had the good fortune to be appointed a member of the school inspectorate, and so not only acquired a firsthand knowledge of the schools, teachers, and pupils, but enjoyed full authority to interrupt the timetable, examine private records, and requisition whatever information might be wanted. Here therefore I must again record my indebtedness both to the London County Council for facilitating these inquiries and financing their publication, and to the teachers, social workers, and school medical officers, who rendered such wholehearted cooperation in all our investigations. It is to be hoped that other education authorities will in the near future perceive the practical value of systematically organized inquiries of this kind, conducted on an official basis by those who know the schools from inside.

The basic researches must be carried out on children rather than on students or adults. With adults, it is much harder to achieve accurate assessments; innate tendencies are already obscured and overlaid; and detailed family histories difficult to obtain. In allocating adults to appropriate occupations, whether in civil life or in the fighting services, innate capacities are of little consequence, and accordingly tend to be ignored. As a result the severest critics of researches on heredity are generally those whose experience of mental testing has been gained in the adult field. This was manifest during the symposium recently arranged by the Psychological Section of the British Association. Several contributors, for instance, echoed remarks like those of H. E. Jones that "potential investigators should now be advised that the nature-nurture controversy has been shown to be an unproductive field of research" (Carmichael, 1946); and similar conclusions have more recently been voiced by writers like Maddox (1957), Renshaw (1957), and others, who deplore what they call "the resurrection of the nature-nurture controversy" as "wholly anachronistic."

But whether or not this is now the prevailing view among psychologists, it is not the opinion of leading geneticists. Goldschmidt, Snyder, Calvin Hall, and Calvin Stone all deplore the neglect of genetic inquiries by psychologists of the present day. Goldschmidt in particular has criticized "the extreme belief of contemporary psychologists in the power of environment"—a belief which he ascribes to the "doctrine of universal conditioning, which has, until lately, dominated the behaviourist school" (Dunn, 1921). In this country eminent authorities like R. A. Fisher (1919, 1950) and Fraser Roberts (1957) have not only urged the importance of genetic studies for psychology, but have made noteworthy contributions of their own.

Mere statistical inquiries, however, can never suffice. In this country one of the most obvious needs is a series of intensive studies of able boys and girls similar to those already carried out on the backward, the defective, the neurotic, and the delinquent.

The brilliant investigation of 1,000 gifted children, started by Terman and his colleagues over 30 years ago, and so assiduously followed up, furnishes an admirable model (1925, 1954). But nothing like conclusive answers can be given to the questions here raised until far more extensive research has been undertaken on the fundamental problems of psychogenetics. An adequate understanding of the basic processes can be secured only if we start with carefully planned experiments on lowlier creatures, where pure strains can be obtained, breeding controlled, and successive generations more speedily raised. When we know more about the genetics of intelligence in animals, we may be able to construct with greater confidence a more exact hypothesis regarding the transmission of intelligence in man.

### *Social Implications*

After all, the practical importance of the issues involved is so profound and so far-reaching that it would be fatal to dismiss the problem as "unproductive" or "anachronistic" without attempting to settle it one way or the other. No democratic state can afford to pass it by. If in the end the views of the early pioneers should turn out to have been approximately correct—if "innate intelligence varies between limits at least as wide as IQ's of 50 and 150," and if too "the average intelligence of the general population at maturity is little if at all above that of an average child of thirteen or thirteen-and-a-half"—then the bearing of genetic variation on the national and social questions of the present day would be all too obvious.

In our laudable eagerness to improve the lot of our own generation, we have been tempted to close our eyes to the effects of present policy on the generations to come. The over-all efficiency of the citizens who make up a nation or a state must in the last resort depend on what has been called its "chromosomal pool."

Improved environmental amenities can of themselves ensure no lasting results; but the changes in a nation's genetic constitution are likely to prove irreversible. Throughout almost the entire Western world, and to a less extent in other areas as well, the last half-century or so has witnessed radical modifications in the conditions that previously governed marriage and fertility. Increased mobility, enhanced freedom, new means of production, new methods of government, the progressive reduction of the traditional barriers separating different peoples and different social groups, and, in our own country, the recent extensions of the educational ladder, all these transformations are visibly disturbing the stability alike of classes and of races. Almost inevitably they must alter the genetic constitution of what have hitherto been the dominant nations and the dominant stocks within those nations.

From history and from past experience we know full well how changes in the balance between inbreeding and outbreeding[11] can affect the later destinies of populations, remoulding them sometimes for good, sometimes for ill. Geneticists have repeatedly drawn attention to the processes at work, and indicated the need for studying the possible effects of contemporary trends (cf., e.g., Darlington and Mather, 1950, pp. 49ff. and Fisher, 1950, pp. 170ff.). Yet current sociological textbooks seem almost wholly

11. British readers will find it instructive to compare current copies of such works as *Who's Who* with those of (say) 60 years ago, and note the changes in the pedigrees of the British clergy (who in the nineteenth century were probably the most inbred profession in the country) and in the ancestry of members of the British cabinet and Civil Service during that period. The recent work of Ginsberg, Glass, and Moss has shown very plainly how the extension of the educational ladder is altering the composition of the different social groups, though none of the writers has considered the possible genetic consequences. The most illuminating discussion is still that contained in the concluding chapters of Fisher's book on *The Genetical Theory of Natural Selection* (1930), especially Chap. X, "Reproduction in Relation to Social Class."

to ignore them. Surely it is high time that the social psychologist should now take up the question and plan a systematic series of investigations on the intricate but highly important issues involved. May I therefore conclude by endorsing, in the strongest possible terms, the verdict of Stone (Dunn, 1921), quoted by Bingham in the last letter he wrote to me:

> It is a matter of shame and regret that only an amateurish beginning has been made by psychologists in applying modern genetic methods to fundamental study in the nature-nurture area.

And may we hope that in the near future Bingham's "deepest wish" may be fulfilled, and that "a small band of enthusiasts will come forward to explore afresh this urgent and many-sided field of research."

### *References*

Bagley, W. C. *The educational process.* New York: Macmillan, 1912.

Burks, Barbara. *27th Yearbook National Society for the Study of Education,* 1928, *1,* 219.

Burt, C. Experimental tests of general intelligence. *Brit. J. Psychol.,* 1909, *3,* 94–177.

Burt, C. The inheritance of mental characteristics. *Eugen. Rev.,* 1912, *4,* 168–200.

Burt, C. *Annual reports of the psychologist to the London County Council.* London: London County Council, 1914–1931.

Burt, C. *The distribution and relations of educational abilities.* London: P. S. King & Son, 1917.

Burt, C. Is the doctrine of instincts dead? *Brit. J. educ. Psychol.,* 1941, *11,* 155–172; 1943, *13,* 1–16a.

Burt, C. The education of the adolescent: the psychological implications of the Norwood Report. *Brit. J. educ. Psychol.,* 1943, *13,* 126–140b.

Burt, C. Ability and income. *Brit. J. educ. Psychol.*, 1943, *13*, 83–98c.
Burt, C. The differentiation of intellectual ability. *Brit. J. educ. Psychol.*, 1954, *24*, 76–90.
Burt, C. The evidence for the concept of intelligence. *Brit. J. educ. Psychol.*, 1955, *25*, 158–177.
Burt, C., & Howard, M. The multifactorial theory of inheritance and its application to intelligence. *Brit. J. statist. Psychol.*, 1956, *9*, 95–131.
Campbell, F. *Eleven plus and all that.* London: Watts, 1956.
Carmichael, L. (ed.). *Manual of child psychology.* New York: Wiley, 1946.
Darlington, C. D., & Mather, K. *The elements of genetics.* London: Allen & Unwin, 1949.
Darlington, C. D., & Mather, K. *Genes, plants, and people.* London: Allen & Unwin, 1950.
Dunn, L. C. (ed.). *Eugenics in the twentieth century.* New York: Macmillan, 1921.
Fisher, R. A. Correlation between relatives on the supposition of Mendelian inheritance. *Trans. roy. Soc., Edin.*, 1918, *52*, 399–433.
Fisher, R. A. The causes of human variability. *Eugen. Rev.*, 1919, *11*, 213–220.
Fisher, R. A. *The genetical theory of natural selection.* Oxford: Clarendon Press, 1950.
Floud, J. E., Halsey, A. H., & Martin, F. M. *Social class and educational opportunity.* London: Heinemann, 1956.
Freeman, F. N. *Mental tests.* New York: Houghton Mifflin, 1926.
Galton, F. *Hereditary Genius.* London: Macmillan, 1869.
Garnett, M. *Education and world citizenship.* Cambridge: Cambridge Univer. Press, 1921.
Goldschmidt, R. B. *Theoretical genetics.* Berkeley: Univer. California Press, 1955.
Lashley, K. S., & Clark, G. The cytoarchitecture of the cerebral cortex of *Ateles:* a critical examination of architectonic studies. *J. comp. Neurol.*, 1946, *85*, 223–305.
Maddox, H. Nature-nurture balance sheets. *Brit. J. educ. Psychol.*, 1957, *27*, 166–175.
Newman, H. H. *Twins and super-twins.* London: Hutchinson, 1942.
Pearson, K. On a generalized theory of alternative inheritance with special reference to Mendel's laws. *Phil. Trans.*, 1904, *203*, 53–87.

Piaget, J. *The psychology of intelligence*. London: Kegan Paul, 1950.
Reeve, F. C. R., & Waddington, C. H. (eds.). *Quantitative inheritance*. London: H. M. Stationery Office, 1952.
Renshaw, T. Burt's concept of intelligence. *Brit. Psychol. Soc. Bull.*, 1957.
Roberts, J. A. F. *An introduction to medical genetics*. Oxford: Oxford Univer. Press, 1940.
Sholl, D. A. *The organization of the cerebral cortex*. London: Methuen, 1956.
Spearman, C. *Abilities of man*. London: Macmillan, 1927.
Spencer, H. *Principles of psychology*. London: Williams & Norgate, 1870.
Stone, C. P. Methodological resources for the experimental study of innate behaviour as related to environmental factors. *Psychol. Rev.*, 1947, *54*, 342–347.
Tanner, J. M. The inheritance of morphological and physiological traits. In A. Sorsby, *Clinical genetics*. London: Butterworth, 1953.
Terman, L. M. (ed.). *Genetic studies of genius*. Stanford: Stanford Univer. Press, 1925, 1947.
Terman, L. M. The discovery and encouragement of exceptional talent. *Amer. Psychologist*, 1954, *9*, 221–230.
Thorndike, E. L. *Educational psychology*. New York: Teachers College, Columbia University, 1914.
Thurstone, L. L. *The vectors of mind*. Chicago: Univer. Chicago Press, 1935.
Watson, J. B. *Behaviourism*. London: Paul, Trench Trubner, 1931.

# *Edward K. Strong, Jr.* *Satisfactions and Interests*[1]

The topic is "Satisfactions and Interests." During the last 37 years I have learned some things about interests, but I confess I have taken satisfaction for granted—which I think is pretty much what most psychologists have done. The term is employed in everyday language and defined in the dictionary. It plays an important role in all theories of motivation. For over three decades surveys of job satisfaction of employees have been conducted costing thousands of dollars. Nevertheless I am very doubtful if any ten experts would agree on a specific definition of the term.

Years ago I contended that there was "no better criterion of a vocational interest test than that of satisfaction enduring over a period of years" (Strong, 1943, p. 385). I have actually never used satisfaction as a criterion on the ground that there seemed to be no good way to measure it. Such correlations as have been reported between interest scores and satisfaction have been for the most part too low to be of practical significance.

1. This paper is based on the Walter Van Dyke Bingham Memorial Lecture given at the University of Minnesota, April 10, 1958. It was first published in the *American Psychologist,* 1958, vol. 13, no. 8 (August), pp. 449–456.

### *Job Satisfaction and Job Success*

Most people have assumed that job satisfaction or morale contributes to production. It came as a shock to me, as it must have done to many others, to read Brayfield and Crockett's (1955) review of the literature and to learn that there is little or no evidence to support the assumption. In a still more recent review, Herzberg, Mausner, Peterson, and Capwell (1957) report some relationship between morale and production, but in most of the investigations where there were positive relations they were low correlations. Reading these two reviews and that of Viteles (1953) and many of the articles on which these reviews are based leaves one bewildered. Definitions of the key terms are conspicuous by their absence and must differ greatly, judging by the context. Many statements by one writer are contradicted by another.

What is satisfaction? Some say it is a kind of feeling as simple as pleasantness; others contend it is a complex of feeling, emotion, and sensation. If the latter, do the proportions of these three ingredients vary each time? Contrast the satisfaction of eating dinner and resting afterwards with a full stomach with the satisfaction of finding a house to rent after hunting many weary days. The mother tells her daughter as she leaves the home to have a good time and asks when the girl returns: "Did you have a good time?" Is having a good time what is meant by satisfaction?

Employee surveys are called attitude or job satisfaction or morale surveys. The terms are sometimes used synonymously and sometimes not. In the absence of generally accepted definitions it is suggested that job satisfaction be employed when the worker is thought of as an individual and that morale be used when the worker is thought of as a member of a group. Perry defines morale as "a state of mind which characterizes groups of men when they are engaged in some action . . . The essence of it is that the group holds together and holds to its objective, despite events that are calculated to divide and dishearten" (1942). An employee is an individual and a member of one or more groups. It is appropriate to consider both his job satisfaction and his morale. But seemingly there should be some difference in the inventories designed to measure these two attitudes towards one's job. Inventories regarding morale should contain items relative to the man's involvement with his company, his union, and the members of his department. Are the low correlations between production and job satisfaction caused in part at least by inadequate measurement of job satisfaction? Consider briefly how job satisfaction has been measured.

Employee surveys since the pioneer days of Houser have typically consisted of two parts: the first part asking a few questions as to the man's overall satisfaction with his job; the second asking whether he liked or was satisfied with all manner of factors, such as income, supervision, cafeteria, pension system, and so on. A summary of the responses in the first part was supposed to measure the employee's overall satisfaction. Responses to the items in the second part that pertained to each job factor were summarized in order to show how satisfied or dissatisfied employees were regarding the various factors. The purpose of such surveys has been to aid management to improve production by determining the causes of dissatisfaction and by identifying the departments with low morale. Much of the literature is devoted to the causes or job factors presumably associated with dissatisfaction, their relative importance, and what can be done to improve conditions. Surveys have been worthwhile to the extent that management has made intelligent use of the results—which has not always been done.

One reason why job satisfaction inventories do not correlate with production is that the items do not furnish good measures of the specific job factors. In one investigation, for example, four questions were used to measure each of four factors; the intercorrelations among the four items ranged from .39 to .52. A summary of the responses of four such questions can only roughly approximate what they purport to measure.

Even if we had good measures of job factors, which we do not have, some of the factors would not correlate particularly with production. Seemingly, health should be directly related to production. But some employees who suffer from poor health plug along regardless, and other employees absent themselves whenever they have the sniffles. Consider one very simple example of physical condition, that of toothache. If we rate production on a scale of $-3$ to $+3$ (where $-3$ represents absence from work and zero production, and $+3$ represents maximum production) and similarly rate satisfaction-dissatisfaction from toothache (where $-3$ represents such severe pain the man is absent at his dentist, the rating of $-2$ represents a decrease of 2 from normal rating in production, and the rating of $-1$ represents a decrease of 1 from normal production), then we will have a correlation of .42 when 35% of employees have ratings of $-3$, $-2$, and $-1$ in dissatisfaction from toothache. If the percentage of employees so affected drops to 15%, the correlation is .26; if the percentage is further decreased to 10%, the correlation is .20. It is unlikely that the percentage of employees seriously affected by toothache is ever as high as 10%, so that the correlation would be appreciably below .20 although the data were arranged so that there was high correlation between suffering from toothache and decrease in production.

In order to obtain a significant correlation between satisfaction-dissatisfaction and production, we must have a situation where dissatisfaction produces decrease, and satisfaction produces increase, in production; and, furthermore, where a fair percentage of employees rate the factor high or low. It is doubtful if most job factors are so related to production.

Consider a second condition, that of being in love. Here we might obtain very high or very low overall satisfaction-dissatisfaction responses depending upon the current behavior of the loved one. It seems probable that those suffering from this malady, whether satisfied or not, would exhibit decrease in production since the employee's attention would be distracted by daydreaming about last night and what will happen on the next date.

The factor of age has a curvilinear relationship with production. The youngest and oldest employees are more satisfied than those about 30 years of age. The factor of age will reduce the correlation when it is mixed in with other factors.

Those of you who are interested should consider how satisfaction-dissatisfaction relative to each aspect of a job could be related to success on the job and also estimate what percentage of employees would be particularly satisfied or dissatisfied on any one day.

A still more serious difficulty arises when responses to all the items on an inventory are summarized on the assumption that, if job satisfaction is to be measured, all aspects of the job should be taken into account. Here, inadequate measures of each factor are combined without much consideration as to the relationships between the factors—a procedure which makes our statisticians fairly froth at the mouth. A way must be found to consider only those who are really satisfied or dissatisfied with each job factor and to disregard those who don't really care about the factor. In the case of toothache there may be perfect correlation with production among the very few suffering with toothache and zero correlation among the great majority. Data based on all of them will not correlate as high as .10. How can you expect to learn how production is related to satisfaction with the job and with expectation of advancement when people with such attitudes are combined with girls who expect to marry and quit work? We need to develop adequate measures of each factor and determine the relationship to an adequate criterion before attempting a summary of all factors.

One way to discover what a test should measure is to note the nature of its items. Four types of questions are found in survey questionnaires: questions asking for facts, opinions, likings, and satisfactions. The proportions of these types vary greatly among survey inventories.

The evidence is clear that facts and opinions about working conditions are colored by feeling—as is every aspect of behavior. It is therefore appropriate to use fact and opinion questions to indicate feeling. Responses should, however, differ according as one is asked: Does your supervisor treat all alike? Do you like your supervisor? Are you satisfied to work under your supervisor? Most inventories ask many interest questions: "Do you like or dislike this and that?" Considering that the inventory is to measure job satisfaction or morale, it is surprising that there are not more items which ask: "Are you satisfied or not with this and that?" Relatively few items inquire as to the man's involvement with his fellows and the company.

The correlations between job satisfaction and production are low not only because measures of job satisfaction are inadequate but because measures of success on the job are also inadequate. It is well recognized that production is not a complete measure of success on the job. There is possibly no more difficult problem in industrial psychology than the determination of adequate criteria of success. Furthermore, in a surprisingly high proportion of jobs there is no way to measure amount of production, and in many cases where it can be measured, as on an assembly line, the measure is far more a measure of flow of work, determined by management, than it is a reflection of the man's ability and willingness to do the work. It is not surprising that psychologists resort so often to ratings of supervisors as their criterion of success. Psychologists have so far contributed relatively little to this task. I have great faith in the ability of psychologists to develop an adequate test of any specifically defined activity; but, if the activity is not definitely defined, the first step should be to define the activity, not to attempt to devise tests that correlate .20, maybe .30, with something that it is hoped represents the activity. It would seem at the present time that both psychologists and management should concentrate on what is meant by success on a given job. When that is accomplished, management ought to be able to measure success on the job, and psychologists should aid in the analyses and devise tests which will predict in advance who will be successful and, I hope, also who will be interested and reasonably satisfied.

What shall be done with job surveys? Three alternatives are evident. First, continue the surveys for their practical value to business management but discontinue trying to prove that morale increases production appreciably. Second, accept the necessity of morale for its own sake. Modern personnel practice stresses that men must be selected so as to be both useful and happy. Maybe we should assume that good morale means general contentment, happiness, satisfaction on the part of all, top management as well as employees. No instructor, supervisor, or army officer wants the people under him to be complaining and criticizing everything that has to be done. Third, develop adequate measures of morale and success on the job. If there were adequate measures, might there not be much higher correlations between them?

Unquestionably much has been learned from job satisfaction surveys of practical use to business and of theoretical value to psychology. It is doubtful, however, if additional surveys will add much more of theoretical value. It now seems highly desirable to isolate and define the basic components and find some way to measure each of them. These are problems for psychologists to tackle. They are not easy or we would know more about them than we do today.

### *Opinion, Attitude, Interest, and Satisfaction*

Consider now four basic concepts: opinion, attitude, interest, and satisfaction. First, what is *opinion*, often referred to as attitude? An opinion is a mental reaction to the relationship between this and that. Many items in an employee survey are opinion items, such as: "Do you work better on a clear or rainy day?" Responses to the questions are either "Yes" or "No" based on facts, more or less, but primarily indicating belief or disbelief. Belief is a feeling comparable to pleasantness, liking, and satisfaction. Opinions concerning religion and membership in the Republican or Democratic party are about as stable as anything we have in life. But many judgments are based on conversation, hearsay, no personal experience, and change about as readily as styles. The hullabaloo following the appearance of Sputnik is a striking example of a whole country losing faith in what they had previously believed. Because opinion items are not as stable as interest items, it is doubtful that they can be as useful as interest items in predicting future behavior. Research is needed to answer this and many other related problems well set forth by Sherif and Cantril (1945) and by McNemar (1946).

A second term is *attitude*. This term has a great vogue today. But what does it signify? Nelson (1939) lists 23 rather distinct characterizations of the term. Sherif and Cantril tell us the term is in a very confused state, and McNemar reminds us that "no one has ever seen an attitude." Seemingly its best usefulness is its ambiguity. When a psychologist does not want to disclose his real purpose, as is typically the case with employee surveys, he may call his inventory a job attitude survey.

Several have given definitions of attitude. Peak's definition of attitude is useful here. She defines attitude (1955) as "a hypothetical construct which involves organization around a conceptual or perceptual nucleus *and* which has affective properties." Concepts and percepts are acquired reactions to a combination of sensations. They are mental activities, and most of them initiate overt activities. It is not merely that sensations are organized into a concept so that no two persons have exactly the same concept but that such concepts are *used* in some manner that is important. What happens when I say the word "baseball"? Do you see the word, or think of keeping score, as you used to do in high school, or do you think of watching a game, or of playing the game, of playing short stop, or knocking out a home run? If the concept is emphasized, then according to Peak we have an attitude; if the activity is emphasized, we have a habit, a skill, or an interest. Psychologists are prone to call activities by many names depending upon the aspect that is emphasized. Thus the activity of skating is called a habit or a skill when its motor coordination acquired by repetition is emphasized; it is called an interest when its feeling quality is emphasized.

Five characteristics of *interests* may be mentioned. First, they are acquired in the sense that feeling becomes associated with the activity. We are not referring to the learning of an activity itself, such as writing one's name, which usually requires many repetitions. We are referring to the associating of feeling with an activity. Such association results from one or only a few experiences—once stung by a bee, one dislikes bees the rest of his life. About all that can be said about the associating process is that, when an activity is useful, aids in reaching some goal, pleasant feeling is attached to it; when the activity is not useful, brings some disagreeable consequence, unpleasant feeling is attached.

Second, interests are persistent. Sometimes disliking is replaced by liking and vice versa; many start out disliking olives and acquire a taste, a pleasant feeling, for them. But, all in all, interests are surprisingly permanent.

A third characteristic of interests is intensity. One can not only immediately indicate whether he likes or dislikes an activity, but one can also immediately indicate his relative preferences for different activities.

The fourth and fifth characteristics are acceptance-rejection and readiness to act. For example, the waitress says: "Will you have some garlic bread?" My wife's response is, "Yes, please"; my own response is, "No, thanks." She likes garlic and goes toward it, I dislike garlic and reject it. Such acceptance-rejection implies action, direction, choice. Such preferences typify readiness to act in the sense that a habit or memory is a readiness to act. The query of the waitress is a stimulus, and the already acquired interest, habit, memory, whatever one wants to call it, functions. The associated value, or feeling quality, determines whether the activity will be accepted or rejected, whether the organism will go toward or away from it, whether it will continue the status quo or discontinue it. It must also be noted that many activities develop in time so as to bring sufficient pleasure to be employed for their own sake. So we smoke, chew gum, play bridge, or golf for the fun of it.

It is not surprising that interest tests predict the direction in which a person will go, for each item is indicative of preference, choice, direction to go. Interest tests are diagnostic because no two persons have acquired the same list of activities nor are the activities classified in the same manner as liked or disliked. Moreover, people engaged in an occupation have to a marked degree similar interests, and so people in one occupation can be differentiated from the members of other occupations.

How shall *satisfaction* be defined? Here again there are many definitions of satisfaction, but most of them emphasize three aspects: first, arrival at a goal, Webster says "fulfillment of a need or desire"; second, pleasant feeling or contentment; and third, a relatively quiescent condition. A sleepy cat purring on a rug, or contented cows, come to mind. But satisfaction occurs not merely when the goal is reached but also long before. These two satisfactions may be referred to as actual and anticipated satisfaction. Anticipation of one's date next Friday night is often much more exciting than the actuality.

Dissatisfaction is the opposite of satisfaction as far as feeling goes, but the overt activities accompanying satisfaction and dissatisfaction are quite different. In the case of actual satisfaction, the series of activities has been completed or nearly so, tension is released, and quiescence follows. In the case of anticipated satisfaction, activities may continue for years, as in the case of the boy planning to be a physician. Here is long range planning, continuing effort. Dissatisfaction arises because the individual is prevented from reaching his goal. He must find some way to circumvent the obstacle, or he must forego his desire. Any interference with one's purpose is frustrating with release of energy and anger. Such explosive behavior is very different from the quiescence of reaching a goal or the long term planning associated with anticipated satisfaction. Expressed in another way, anticipated satisfaction accompanies progress toward a goal, while dissatisfaction arises when progress is prevented.

I have had a lot of fun asking my colleagues what is the difference between interests and satisfactions. They start out quite sure they know and often end up quite confused. One distinction is that interests are associated with activities, and satisfactions are not. It is true that there are certain activities regularly employed to satisfy bodily needs, but the striking characteristic in securing satisfaction is that one uses whatever activities are available and may use a different combination of activities each time a goal is sought. Aside from the final, consummatory activity, satisfaction cannot be identified in terms of activities, as can interests.

Can interests and satisfactions be differentiated in terms of feeling? Interests are liked or disliked; there seems to be no qualitative difference in the liking of different activities. Satisfactions of bodily needs differ in quality. But possibly this is so because of the presence of different sensations. If the sensations were eliminated, would the remaining satisfactions be similar in such cases? What about goals other than bodily needs? Are there qualitative differences in the satisfactions of earning an *A* grade, in winning the high jump, in finding a house to rent, and so on? On the negative side, disliked activities tend to be ignored. But if one is forced to employ a disliked activity, as fixing a flat tire, the reaction is more typically dissatisfaction than disliking; then one grumbles, complains, swears, and even exhibits all the symptoms of anger.

Finally how can satisfaction-dissatisfaction be measured? We have already mentioned how job satisfaction is measured and that improvements are greatly needed before adequate measurements can be obtained as to how much satisfaction-dissatisfaction is associated with each job factor. Before considering a different procedure, let us eliminate measurement of satisfaction-dissatisfaction of past events on the grounds that they cannot be measured with any accuracy; and even if they could, they would be of little value.

A man who liked to fish and to golf but no longer does so because of old age continues to say he likes such activities. It is possible that, if he were asked to arrange a long list of activities in order of preference, he would not rank fishing and golf as high as he would have done 20 years earlier. Nevertheless he still likes them. The question is: Can one feel satisfaction for past events in similar fashion? I once hiked through heavy brush in hot weather for over 24 hours without food or water. It must have been very rugged, but I cannot now conjure up the thirst and fatigue I must have experienced. I can only recall the incident and enjoy talking about it as I am doing now. My old friend Hollingworth would have exclaimed: "That exemplifies the oblivescence of the disagreeable." My present feeling of pleasure at having done it is very different from how I must have felt at the time. Consider another incident. A violent argument arises in the machine shop as to how a job is to be done. The man who wins feels satisfied, the other dissatisfied. Now, if as so often happens the incident is forgotten the next day and there is no bad feeling on either side, then there is no existing satisfaction or dissatisfaction. And if so, is there any value today in trying to measure the feelings of yesterday? But if the loser in the argument continues to be sore, then such existing dissatisfaction may have a bearing on his overall satisfaction-dissatisfaction.

What about satisfaction-dissatisfaction concerning a goal not yet attained? Here three components are evident: the goal, the dissatisfaction of today, and the anticipated satisfaction of tomorrow. The difference between the last two is, however, more significant than either, or both, considered separately.

In attempting to explain persistence of motivation Peak suggests that it is the "discrepancy rather than the affect which is the important source of continuing action." It is the difference between "Harry's feeling about his present job . . . and his feeling for the ideal job that he imagines" that is the source of persistent efforts to achieve the ideal. This agrees with what I have long taught: that motivation, or "intensifying the want of a prospect in selling, involves, first, making him realize how unpleasant his present situation is, and second, making him anticipate as much as possible the enjoyment he will have when he reaches his desired goal" (1938). Morse (1953) has this same conception in mind when she says that "satisfaction depends basically upon what an individual wants from the world and what he gets." We would suggest substituting what "he expects to get" for "what he gets."

### *Measurement of Motivation*

What we are proposing is the measurement of motivation rather than satisfaction of a given moment. Motivation is a more dynamic aspect of behavior than satisfaction and should prove more useful in predicting future behavior. It is worthwhile to know how an employee feels towards this or that right now, today. But it is more important to know whether he is going to continue in his present type of work, to continue with the company, or to do something else. Job surveys have asked: "How satisfied are you with this and that?" In contrast we ask: "What do you want?" "What do you expect to get?" and "What do you think are the chances you will get what you want?" The difference between aspiration and expectation affords a basis of estimating degree of dissatisfaction; but likelihood that the expectation will be achieved must also be taken into account. The greater the expectation, the greater is the anticipated satisfaction.

It should be noted in passing that measurement of motivation is similar to measurement of interests in that neither predicts how far or how fast one will go, for success is primarily a matter of ability, but both indicate direction, which of many activities will be engaged in.

Specific goals must be considered as well as present dissatisfaction and anticipated satisfaction. It is futile to compare the feelings of a girl who is working hard to make good and become office manager with those of a girl who is planning to quit work, marry, and have a home of her own, even though at the moment they are both dissatisfied with their progress toward their different goals.

Goals are phantasies, wishes, daydreams, aspirations, plans.

Goals are often called needs. Some of them are needs but most have evolved as the result of social pressures, often expressed as "Keeping up with the Joneses." Many of these seem imperative, but does one have to keep up with the Joneses in every respect?

Have we any idea how many different goals the men and women in this country possess, if all were expressed in standard terminology? Does a given man possess during his lifetime all possible goals or only a few? If the latter, why has he these particular goals? Again, how many goals does a man have at a given time? It is also important to know whether each goal is accompanied by its own satisfaction-dissatisfaction quality or do all these qualities more or less fuse together? In other words, does unhappiness because of one's wife affect one's attitude toward one's job, and vice versa? Does the dissatisfaction at being fired from one's job and the satisfaction from one's girl's promise to marry him alternate so that he fluctuates from dissatisfaction to satisfaction; or do the two fuse, and if so is the fusion a mere average or a weighted average in terms of their relative significance?

Goals differ also in complexity. There are simple goals as getting to class on time and complex goals such as planning to graduate from college while still in high school. Such long distant goals necessitate careful planning in terms of many subgoals, as selecting the courses necessary to enter college, getting good enough grades, selection of a college, etc.

It is necessary to determine not only a man's goals but the chance, the likelihood, of his attaining his goal. Likelihood is dependent here not upon the actual facts but upon the man's opinion or belief. A former student resigned because he saw no future in being moved from one job to another, not knowing that he was being groomed for an important position. The greater the chance, the greater is the anticipating satisfaction; the less the chance, the greater is the dissatisfaction. When there is no chance, the man may quit (a friend of mine committed suicide), or nurse a grudge, or abandon his goal (often not easy to do), or find a substitute goal. Likelihood may be expressed in terms of money as in buying an auto or home; or it may be expressed in terms of effort, that is, practice or study; or in terms of willingness to forego other goals, often called pleasures.

With many goals there is a cycle from dissatisfaction to satisfaction, repeated over and over. A simple example is eating. Three times a day we want to eat, are satisfied, and quit thinking about eating for a short while. Another example pertains to salary. Start with dissatisfaction, then anticipated satisfaction when the grapevine reports there will be raises, then satisfaction when the increase is received, then little thought of the subject gradually changing to dissatisfaction. Answers to the static question, "Are you satisfied with your salary?" depends upon where the man is in such a cycle. The more dynamic questions of: "What salary do you want a year hence, five years hence?" and "What do you think the chances are of obtaining such salaries?" should provide a more forward-looking picture of the man's reaction to his salary. Whether men can look five years ahead or not is something to be determined. A few years ago I tried out such questions with college seniors; the great majority could not or would not give anything like definite answers.

Satisfaction in the long run necessitates improvement, progress. A golfer who had never had a better score than 85 would be elated with 84. But if he had 84 every time for several weeks, he would become steadily more dissatisfied; only an 83 or better would give him satisfaction. Many investigators have pointed out that men about 30 years old are more dissatisfied than younger and older men. Is this not due to the fact that such 30-year-old men have come to realize that future progress is limited, that they are not going to realize their aspirations? Some remain disgruntled, but many seek satisfaction in other activities.

The term "level of aspiration" has considerable vogue today. Presumably it represents fairly well formulated to clear-cut formulation of one's goals. Why does one young man aspire to be a lawyer and his brother follow in the footsteps of his father, a coal miner? We always come back to the old, old problem: did the two go in different directions because of environmental educational pressures or because their genes were different? I have a hunch that many adult goals have evolved out of phantasies and daydreams. A 10-year-old girl dreamed of accompanying Allan Quartermain on wild adventures in Africa; later on she has always said "Yes" to her husband's harum-scarum expeditions. Is there any connection? Why did she indulge in exploration and physical danger instead of being a movie actress, a princess, or a Cinderella? How can one ascertain what daydreams a person has, considering that daydreams are usually viewed as too personal, too self-revealing, to be divulged to anyone? No psychologist will achieve fame by predicting future behavior on the basis of well-formulated plans; the really tough task is to predict behavior in terms of the antecedents of such plans.

I hope it has occurred to you that there are two great problems: What can this person do, what are his abilities, what can he accomplish if his abilities are properly trained; and, second, what does he want to do, which way does he want to go in life? His satisfaction, happiness, contentment is dependent upon the direction he is permitted to go. Happiness and success are interrelated, but all counseling services both educational and industrial must seek reasonable success for their counselees and also happiness now and in the future. Such counseling is dependent upon a determination of capacities on the one hand and goals on the other hand. We have made far more progress in measuring capacities than in ascertaining men's goals.

I have asked many questions for which I don't know the answers. There are hundreds of difficulties in all this—I am tempted to say a million difficulties. A good research man ought not to be dismayed; rather he should glory in the complexities—a tough job is far more fun than an easy one.

### *References*

Brayfield, A. H., & Crockett, W. H. Employee attitudes and employee performance. *Psychol. Bull.*, 1955, *52*, 396–424.

Herzberg, F., Mausner, B., Peterson, R. O., & Capwell, D. F. *Job attitudes: review of research and opinion.* Pittsburgh: Psychological Services of Pittsburgh, 1957.

McNemar, Q. Opinion-attitude methodology. *Psychol. Bull.*, 1946, *43*, 289–374.

Morse, N. C. *Satisfaction in the white-collar jobs.* Ann Arbor: Institute for Social Research, 1953.

Nelson, E. Attitudes: I. Their nature and development. *J. gen. Psychol.*, 1939, *21*, 367–399.

Peak, H. Attitude and motivation. In *Nebraska symposium on motivation*, 1955.

Perry, R. B. National morale. *Educ. Rec.*, 1942, *23*, Suppl. No. 15.

Sherif, M., & Cantril, H. The psychology of attitudes. Part I. *Psychol. Rev.*, 1945, *52*, 295–319.

Strong, E. K., Jr. *Psychological aspects of business.* New York: McGraw-Hill, 1938.

Strong, E. K., Jr. *Vocational interests of men and women.* Stanford: Stanford Univer. Press, 1943.

Viteles, M. S. *Motivation and morale in industry.* New York: Norton, 1953.

# *J. P. Guilford* *Three Faces of Intellect*[1]

My subject is in the area of human intelligence, in connection with which the names of Terman and Stanford have become known the world over. The Stanford Revision of the Binet intelligence scale has been the standard against which all other instruments for the measurement of intelligence have been compared. The term IQ or intelligence quotient has become a household word in this country. This is illustrated by two brief stories.

> A few years ago, one of my neighbors came home from a PTA meeting, remarking: "That Mrs. So-And-So, thinks she knows so much. She kept talking about the 'intelligence *quota*' of the children; 'intelligence *quota*'; imagine. Why, everybody knows that IQ stands for 'intelligence *quiz*.'"
>
> The other story comes from a little comic strip in a Los Angeles morning newspaper, called "Junior Grade." In the first picture a little boy meets a little girl, both apparently about the first-grade level. The little girl remarks, "I have

1. This paper is based on the Walter Van Dyke Bingham Memorial Lecture given at Stanford University, April 13, 1959. It was first published in the *American Psychologist*, 1959, vol. 14, no. 8 (August), pp. 469–479.

a high IQ." The little boy, puzzled, said, "You have a what?" The little girl repeated, "I have a high IQ," then went on her way. The little boy, looking thoughtful, said, "And she looks like such a nice little girl, too."

It is my purpose to speak about the analysis of this thing called human intelligence into its components. I do not believe that either Binet or Terman, if they were still with us, would object to the idea of a searching and detailed study of intelligence, aimed toward a better understanding of its nature. Preceding the development of his intelligence scale, Binet had done much research on different kinds of thinking activities and apparently recognized that intelligence has a number of aspects. It is to the lasting credit of both Binet and Terman that they introduced such a great variety of tasks into their intelligence scales.

Two related events of very recent history make it imperative that we learn all we can regarding the nature of intelligence. I am referring to the advent of the artificial satellites and planets and to the crisis in education that has arisen in part as a consequence. The preservation of our way of life and our future security depend upon our most important national resources: our intellectual abilities and, more particularly, our creative abilities. It is time, then, that we learn all we can about those resources.

Our knowledge of the components of human intelligence has come about mostly within the last 25 years. The major sources of this information in this country have been L. L. Thurstone and his associates, the wartime research of psychologists in the United States Air Force, and more recently the Aptitudes Project[2] at the University of Southern California, now in its tenth year of research on cognitive and thinking abilities. The results from the Aptitudes Project that have gained perhaps the most atten-

2. Under Contract N6onr-23810 with the Office of Naval Research (Personnel and Training Branch).

tion have pertained to creative-thinking abilities. These are mostly novel findings. But to me, the most significant outcome has been the development of a unified theory of human intellect, which organizes the known, unique or primary intellectual abilities into a single system called the "structure of intellect." It is to this system that I shall devote the major part of my remarks, with very brief mentions of some of the implications for the psychology of thinking and problem solving, for vocational testing, and for education.

The discovery of the components of intelligence has been by means of the experimental application of the method of factor analysis. It is not necessary for you to know anything about the theory or method of factor analysis in order to follow the discussion of the components. I should like to say, however, that factor analysis has no connection with or resemblance to psychoanalysis. A positive statement would be more helpful, so I will say that each intellectual component or factor is a unique ability that is needed to do well in a certain class of tasks or tests. As a general principle we find that certain individuals do well in the tests of a certain class, but they may do poorly in the tests of another class. We conclude that a factor has certain properties from the features that the tests of a class have in common. I shall give you very soon a number of examples of tests, each representing a factor.

### *The Structure of Intellect*

Although each factor is sufficiently distinct to be detected by factor analysis, in very recent years it has become apparent that the factors themselves can be classified because they resemble one another in certain ways. One basis of classification is according to the basic kind of process or operation performed. This kind of classification gives us five major groups of intellectual abilities: factors of cognition, memory, convergent thinking, divergent thinking, and evaluation.

Cognition means discovery or rediscovery or recognition. Memory means retention of what is cognized. Two kinds of productive-thinking operations generate new information from known information and remembered information. In divergent-thinking operations we think in different directions, sometimes searching, sometimes seeking variety. In convergent thinking the information leads to one right answer or to a recognized best or conventional answer. In evaluation we reach decisions as to goodness, correctness, suitability, or adequacy of what we know, what we remember, and what we produce in productive thinking.

A second way of classifying the intellectual factors is according to the kind of material or content involved. The factors known thus far involve three kinds of material or content: the content may be figural, symbolic, or semantic. Figural content is concrete material such as is perceived through the senses. It does not represent anything except itself. Visual material has properties such as size, form, color, location, or texture. Things we hear or feel provide other examples of figural material. Symbolic content is composed of letters, digits, and other conventional signs, usually organized in general systems, such as the alphabet or the number sytem. Semantic content is in the form of verbal meanings or ideas, for which no examples are necessary.

When a certain operation is applied to a certain kind of content, as many as six general kinds of products may be involved. There is enough evidence available to suggest that, regardless of the combinations of operations and content, the same six kinds of products may be found associated. The six kinds of products are: units, classes, relations, systems, transformations, and implications. So far as we have determined from factor analysis, these are the only fundamental kinds of products that we can know. As such, they may serve as basic classes into which one might fit all kinds of information psychologically.

The three kinds of classifications of the factors of intellect can be represented by means of a single solid model, shown in Figure 1. In this model, which we call the "structure of intellect," each dimension represents one of the modes of variation of the

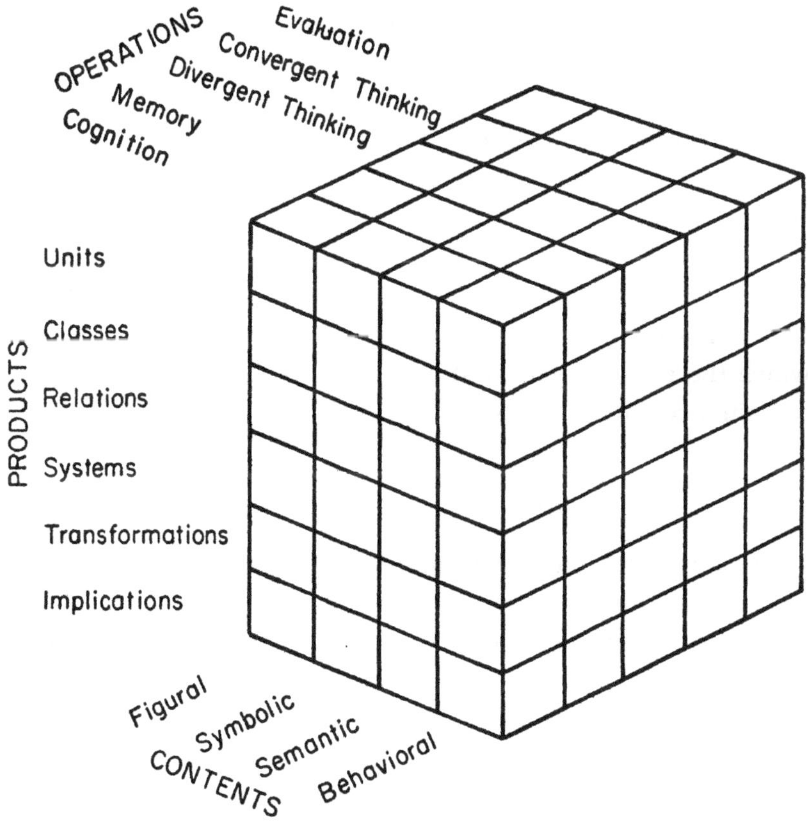


Fig. 1. A cubical model representing the structure of intellect.

factors.[3] Along one dimension are found the various kinds of operations, along a second one are the various kinds of products, and along the third are various kinds of content. Along the dimension of content a fourth category has been added, its kind of content being designated as "behavioral." This category has been added on a purely theoretical basis to represent the general area sometimes called "social intelligence." More will be said about this section of the model later.

In order to provide a better basis for understanding the model and a better basis for accepting it as a picture of human intellect, I shall do some exploring of it with you systematically, giving some examples of tests. Each cell in the model calls for a certain kind of ability that can be described in terms of operation, content, and product, for each cell is at the intersection of a unique combination of kinds of operation, content, and product. A test for that ability would have the same three properties. In our exploration of the model, we shall take one vertical layer at a time, beginning with the front face. The first layer provides us with a matrix of 18 cells (if we ignore the behavioral column for which there are as yet no known factors) each of which should contain a cognitive ability.

### *The Cognitive Abilities*

We know at present the unique abilities that fit logically into 15 of the 18 cells for cognitive abilities. Each row presents a triad of similar abilities, having a single kind of product in common. The factors of the first row are concerned with the knowing of units. A good test of the ability to cognize figural units is the Street Gestalt Completion Test. In this test, the recognition of familiar pictured objects in silhouette form is made difficult for

3. For an earlier presentation of the concept, see Guilford (1956).

testing purposes by blocking out parts of those objects. There is another factor that is known to involve the perception of auditory figures—in the form of melodies, rhythms, and speech sounds—and still another factor involving kinesthetic forms. The presence of three factors in one cell (they are conceivably distinct abilities, although this has not been tested) suggests that more generally, in the figural column, at least, we should expect to find more than one ability. A fourth dimension pertaining to variations in sense modality may thus apply in connection with figural content. The model could be extended in this manner if the facts call for such an extension.

The ability to cognize symbolic units is measured by tests like the following:

Put vowels in the following blanks to make real words:

P__W__R
M__RV__L
C__RT__N

Rearrange the letters to make real words:

RACIH
TVOES
KLCCO

The first of these two tests is called Disemvoweled Words, and the second Scrambled Words.

The ability to cognize semantic units is the well-known factor of verbal comprehension, which is best measured by means of a vocabulary test, with items such as:

GRAVITY means ______
CIRCUS means ______
VIRTUE means ______

From the comparison of these two factors it is obvious that recognizing familiar words as letter structures and knowing what words mean depend upon quite different abilities.

For testing the abilities to know classes of units, we may present the following kinds of items, one with symbolic content and one with semantic content:

Which letter group does not belong?
XECM PVAA QXIN VTRO

Which object does not belong?
clam tree oven rose

A figural test is constructed in a completely parallel form, presenting in each item four figures, three of which have a property in common and the fourth lacking that property.

The three abilities to see relationships are also readily measured by a common kind of test, differing only in terms of content. The well-known analogies test is applicable, two items in symbolic and semantic form being:

| | | | | | | | | | | | | |
|---|---|---|---|---|---|---|---|---|---|---|---|---|
| JIRE | : | KIRE | : | : | FORA | : | KORE | KORA | LIRE | GORA | GIRE |
| poetry | : | prose | : | : | dance | : | music | walk | sing | talk | jump |

Such tests usually involve more than the ability to cognize relations, but we are not concerned with this problem at this point.

The three factors for cognizing systems do not at present appear in tests so closely resembling one another as in the case of the examples just given. There is nevertheless an underlying common core of logical similarity. Ordinary space tests, such as Thurstone's Flags, Figures, and Cards or Part V (Spatial Orientation) of the Guilford-Zimmerman Aptitude Survey (GZAS), serve in the figural column. The system involved is an order or arrangement of objects in space. A system that uses symbolic elements is illustrated by the Letter Triangle Test, a sample item of which is:

___<br>
d ___<br>
b e ___<br>
a c f ?

What letter belongs at the place of the question mark?

The ability to understand a semantic system has been known for some time as the factor called general reasoning. One of its most faithful indicators is a test composed of arithmetic-reasoning items. That the phase of understanding only is important for measuring this ability is shown by the fact that such a test works even if the examinee is not asked to give a complete solution; he need only show that he structures the problem properly. For example, an item from the test Necessary Arithmetical Operations simply asks what operations are needed to solve the problem:

A city lot 48 feet wide and 149 feet deep costs $79,432. What is the cost per square foot?

A. add and multiply
B. multiply and divide
C. subtract and divide
D. add and subtract
E. divide and add

Placing the factor of general reasoning in this cell of the structure of intellect gives us some new conceptions of its nature. It should be a broad ability to grasp all kinds of systems that are conceived in terms of verbal concepts, not restricted to the understanding of problems of an arithmetical type.

Transformations are changes of various kinds, including modifications in arrangement, organization, or meaning. In the figural column for the transformations row, we find the factor known as visualization. Common measuring instruments for this factor are the surface-development tests, and an example of a different kind is Part VI (Spatial Visualization) of the GZAS. A test of the ability to make transformations of meaning, for the factor in the semantic column, is called Similarities. The examinee is asked to state several ways in which two objects, such as an apple and an orange, are alike. Only by shifting the meanings of both is the examinee able to give many responses to such an item.

In the set of abilities having to do with the cognition of implications, we find that the individual goes beyond the information given, but not to the extent of what might be called drawing conclusions. We may say that he extrapolates. From the given information he expects or foresees certain consequences, for example. The two factors found in this row of the cognition matrix were first called "foresight" factors. Foresight in connection with figural material can be tested by means of paper-and-pencil mazes. Foresight in connection with ideas, those pertaining to events, for example, is indicated by a test such as Pertinent Questions:

> In planning to open a new hamburger stand in a certain community, what four questions should be considered in deciding upon its location?

The more questions the examinee asks in response to a list of such problems, the more he evidently foresees contingencies.

### *The Memory Abilities*

The area of memory abilities has been explored less than some of the other areas of operation, and only seven of the potential cells of the memory matrix have known factors in them. These cells are restricted to three rows: for units, relations, and systems. The first cell in the memory matrix is now occupied by two factors, parallel to two in the corresponding cognition matrix: visual memory and auditory memory. Memory for series of letters or numbers, as in memory span tests, conforms to the conception of memory for symbolic units. Memory for the ideas in a paragraph conforms to the conception of memory for semantic units.

The formation of associations between units, such as visual forms, syllables, and meaningful words, as in the method of paired associates, would seem to represent three abilities to remember relationships involving three kinds of content. We know of two such abilities, for the symbolic and semantic columns. The memory for known systems is represented by two abilities very recently discovered (Christal, 1958). Remembering the arrangement of objects in space is the nature of an ability in the figural column, and remembering a sequence of events is the nature of a corresponding ability in the semantic column. The differentiation between these two abilities implies that a person may be able to say where he saw an object on a page, but he might not be able to say on which of several pages he saw it after leafing through several pages that included the right one. Considering the blank rows in the memory matrix, we should expect to find abilities also to remember classes, transformations, and implications, as well as units, relations, and systems.

### *The Divergent-Thinking Abilities*

The unique feature of divergent production is that a *variety* of responses is produced. The product is not completely determined by the given information. This is not to say that divergent thinking does not come into play in the total process of reaching a unique conclusion, for it comes into play wherever there is trial-and-error thinking.

The well-known ability of word fluency is tested by asking the examinee to list words satisfying a specified letter requirement, such as words beginning with the letter "s" or words ending in "-tion." This ability is now regarded as a facility in divergent production of symbolic units. The parallel semantic ability has been known as ideational fluency. A typical test item calls for listing objects that are round and edible. Winston Churchill must have possessed this ability to a high degree. Clement Attlee is reported to have said about him recently that, no matter what problem came up, Churchill always seemed to have about ten ideas. The trouble was, Attlee continued, he did not know which was the good one. The last comment implies some weakness in one or more of the evaluative abilities.

The divergent production of class ideas is believed to be the unique feature of a factor called "spontaneous flexibility." A typical test instructs the examinee to list all the uses he can think of for a common brick, and he is given eight minutes. If his responses are: build a house, build a barn, build a garage, build a school, build a church, build a chimney, build a walk, and build a barbecue, he would earn a fairly high score for ideational fluency but a very low score for spontaneous flexibility, because all these uses fall into the same class. If another person said: make a door stop, make a paper weight, throw it at a dog, make a bookcase, drown a cat, drive a nail, make a red powder, and use for baseball bases, he would also receive a high score for flexibility. He has gone frequently from one class to another.

A current study of unknown but predicted divergent-production abilities includes testing whether there are also figural and symbolic abilities to produce multiple classes. An experimental figural test presents a number of figures that can be classified in groups of three in various ways, each figure being usable in more than one class. An experimental symbolic test presents a few numbers that are also to be classified in multiple ways.

A unique ability involving relations is called "associational fluency." It calls for the production of a variety of things related in a specified way to a given thing. For example, the examinee is asked to list words meaning about the same as "good" or to list words meaning about the opposite of "hard." In these instances the response produced is to complete a relationship, and semantic content is involved. Some of our present experimental tests call for the production of varieties of relations, as such, and involve figural and symbolic content also. For example, given four small digits, in how many ways can they be related in order to produce a sum of eight?

One factor pertaining to the production of systems is known as expressional fluency. The rapid formation of phrases or sentences is the essence of certain tests of this factor. For example, given the initial letters:

W____ c____ e____ n____

with different sentences to be produced, the examinee might write "We can eat nuts" or "Whence came Eve Newton?" In interpreting the factor, we regard the sentence as a symbolic system. By analogy, a figural system would be some kind of organization of lines and other elements, and a semantic system would be in the form of a verbally stated problem or perhaps something as complex as a theory.

In the row of the divergent-production matrix devoted to transformations, we find some very interesting factors. The one called "adaptive flexibility" is now recognized as belonging in the figural column. A faithful test of it has been Match Problems. This is based upon the common game that uses squares, the sides of which are formed by match sticks. The examinee is told to take away a given number of matches to leave a stated number of squares with nothing left over. Nothing is said about the sizes of the squares to be left. If the examinee imposes upon himself the restriction that the squares that he leaves must be of the same size, he will fail in his attempts to do items like that in Figure 2. Other odd kinds of solutions are introduced in other items, such as overlapping squares and squares within squares, and so on. In another variation of Match Problems the examinee is told to produce two or more solutions for each problem.

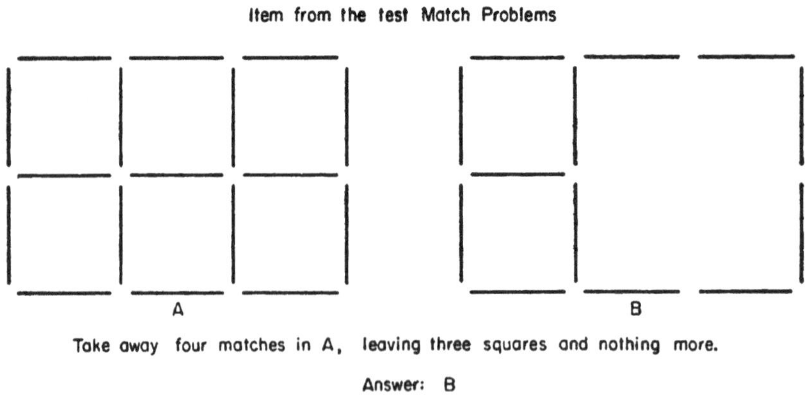


Fig. 2. A sample item from the test Match Problems. The problem in this item is to take away four matches and leave three squares. The solution is given.

A factor that has been called "originality" is now recognized as adaptive flexibility with semantic material, where there must be a shifting of meanings. The examinee must produce the shifts or changes in meaning and so come up with novel, unusual, clever, or farfetched ideas. The Plot Titles Test presents a short story, the examinee being told to list as many appropriate titles as he can to head the story. One story is about a missionary who has been captured by cannibals in Africa. He is in the pot and about to be boiled when a princess of the tribe obtains a promise for his release if he will become her mate. He refuses and is boiled to death.

In scoring the test, we separate the responses into two categories, clever and nonclever. Examples of nonclever responses are: African Death, Defeat of a Princess, Eaten by Savages, The Princess, The African Missionary, In Darkest Africa, and Boiled by Savages. These titles are appropriate but commonplace. The number of such responses serves as a score for ideational fluency. Examples of clever responses are: Pot's Plot, Potluck Dinner, Stewed Parson, Goil or Boil, A Mate Worse Than Death, He Left a Dish for a Pot, Chaste in Haste, and A Hot Price for Freedom. The number of clever responses given by an examinee is his score for originality, or the divergent production of semantic transformations.

Another test of originality presents a very novel task so that any acceptable response is unusual for the individual. In the Symbol Production Test the examinee is to produce a simple symbol to stand for a noun or a verb in each short sentence, in other words to invent something like pictographic symbols. Still another test of originality asks for writing the "punch lines" for cartoons, a task that almost automatically challenges the examinee to be clever. Thus, quite a variety of tests offer approaches to the measurement of originality, including one or two others that I have not mentioned.

Abilities to produce a variety of implications are assessed by tests calling for elaboration of given information. A figural test of this type provides the examinee with a line or two, to which he is to add other lines to produce an object. The more lines he adds, the greater his score. A semantic test gives the examinee the outlines of a plan to which he is to respond by stating all the details he can think of to make the plan work. A new test we are trying out in the symbolic area presents two simple equations such as $B - C = D$ and $z = A + D$. The examinee is to make as many other equations as he can from this information.

## *The Convergent-Production Abilities*

Of the 18 convergent-production abilities expected in the three content columns, 12 are now recognized. In the first row, pertaining to units, we have an ability to name figural properties (forms or colors) and an ability to name abstractions (classes, relations, and so on). It may be that the ability in common to the speed of naming forms and the speed of naming colors is not appropriately placed in the convergent-thinking matrix. One might expect that the thing to be produced in a test of the convergent production of figural units would be in the form of figures rather than words. A better test of such an ability might somehow specify the need for one particular object, the examinee to furnish the object.

A test for the convergent production of classes (Word Grouping) presents a list of 12 words that are to be classified in four, and only four, meaningful groups, no word to appear in more than one group. A parallel test (Figure Concepts Test) presents 20 pictured real objects that are to be grouped in meaningful classes of two or more each.

Convergent production having to do with relationships is represented by three known factors, all involving the "education of correlates," as Spearman called it. The given information includes one unit and a stated relation, the examinee to supply the other unit. Analogies tests that call for completion rather than a choice between alternative answers emphasize this kind of ability. With symbolic content such an item might read:

pots stop    bard drab    rats ?

A semantic item that measures eduction of correlates is:

The absence of sound is ______.

Incidentally, the latter item is from a vocabulary-completion test, and its relation to the factor of ability to produce correlates indicates how, by change of form, a vocabulary test may indicate an ability other than that for which vocabulary tests are usually intended, namely, the factor of verbal comprehension.

Only one factor for convergent production of systems is known, and it is in the semantic column. It is measured by a class of tests that may be called ordering tests. The examinee may be presented with a number of events that ordinarily have a best or most logical order, the events being presented in scrambled order. The presentation may be pictorial, as in the Picture Arrangement Test, or verbal. The pictures may be taken from a cartoon strip. The verbally presented events may be in the form of the various steps needed to plant a new lawn. There are undoubtedly other kinds of systems than temporal order that could be utilized for testing abilities in this row of the convergent-production matrix.

In the way of producing transformations of a unique variety, we have three recognized factors, known as redefinition abilities. In each case, redefinition involves the changing of functions or uses of parts of one unit and giving them new functions or uses in some new unit. For testing the ability of figural redefinition, a task based upon the Gottschaldt figures is suitable. Figure 3 shows the kind of item for such a test. In recognizing the simpler figure within the structure of a more complex figure, certain lines must take on new roles.

In terms of symbolic material, the following sample items will illustrate how groups of letters in given words must be readapted

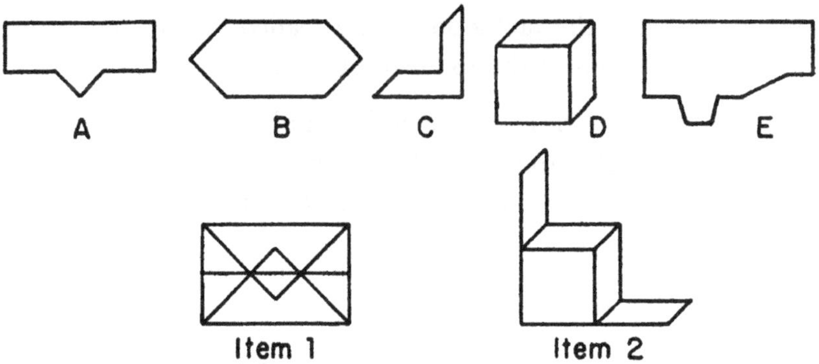


Fig. 3. Sample items from a test Hidden Figures, based upon the Gottschaldt figures. Which of the simpler figures is concealed within each of the two more complex figures?

to use in other words. In the test Camouflaged Words, each sentence contains the name of a sport or game:

> I did not know that he was ailing.
> To beat the Hun, tin goes a long way.

For the factor of semantic redefinition, the Gestalt Transformation Test may be used. A sample item reads:

> From which object could you most likely make a needle?
>
> A. a cabbage
> B. a splice
> C. a steak
> D. a paper box
> E. a fish

The convergent production of implications means the drawing of fully determined conclusions from given information. The well-known factor of numerical facility belongs in the symbolic column. For the parallel ability in the figural column, we have a test known as Form Reasoning, in which rigorously defined operations with figures are used. For the parallel ability in the semantic column, the factor sometimes called "deduction" probably qualifies. Items of the following type are sometimes used.

> Charles is younger than Robert
> Charles is older than Frank
> Who is older: Robert or Frank?

### *Evaluative Abilities*

The evaluative area has had the least investigation of all the operational categories. In fact, only one systematic analytical study has been devoted to this area. Only eight evaluative abilities are recognized as fitting into the evaluation matrix. But at least five rows have one or more factors each, and also three of the usual columns or content categories. In each case, evaluation involves reaching decisions as to the accuracy, goodness, suitability, or workability of information. In each row, for the particular kind of product of that row, some kind of criterion or standard of judgment is involved.

In the first row, for the evaluation of units, the important decision to be made pertains to the identity of a unit. Is this unit identical with that one? In the figural column we find the factor long known as "perceptual speed." Tests of this factor invariably call for decisions of identity, for example, Part IV (Perceptual Speed) of the GZAS or Thurstone's Identical Forms. I think it has been generally wrongly thought that the ability involved is that of cognition of visual forms. But we have seen that another factor is a more suitable candidate for this definition and for being in the very first cell of the cognitive matrix. It is parallel to this evaluative ability but does not require the judgment of identity as one of its properties.

In the symbolic column is an ability to judge identity of symbolic units, in the form of series of letters or numbers or of names of individuals.

Are members of the following pairs identical or not?

825170493_____825176493
dkeltvmpa_____dkeltvmpa
C. S. Meyerson_____C. E. Meyerson

Such items are common in tests of clerical aptitude.

There should be a parallel ability to decide whether two ideas are identical or different. Is the idea expressed in this sentence the same as the idea expressed in that one? Do these two proverbs express essentially the same idea? Such tests exist and will be used to test the hypothesis that such an ability can be demonstrated.

No evaluative abilities pertaining to classes have as yet been recognized. The abilities having to do with evaluation where relations are concerned must meet the criterion of logical consistency. Syllogistic-type tests involving letter symbols indicate a different ability than the same type of test involving verbal statements. In the figural column we might expect that tests incorporating geometric reasoning or proof would indicate a parallel ability to sense the soundness of conclusions regarding figural relationships.

The evaluation of systems seems to be concerned with the internal consistency of those systems, so far as we can tell from the knowledge of one such factor. The factor has been called "experiential evaluation," and its representative test presents items like that in Figure 4 asking "What is wrong with this picture?" The things wrong are often internal inconsistencies.

A semantic ability for evaluating transformations is thought to be that known for some time as "judgment." In typical judgment tests, the examinee is asked to tell which of five solutions to a practical problem is most adequate or wise. The solutions frequently involve improvisations, in other words, adaptations of

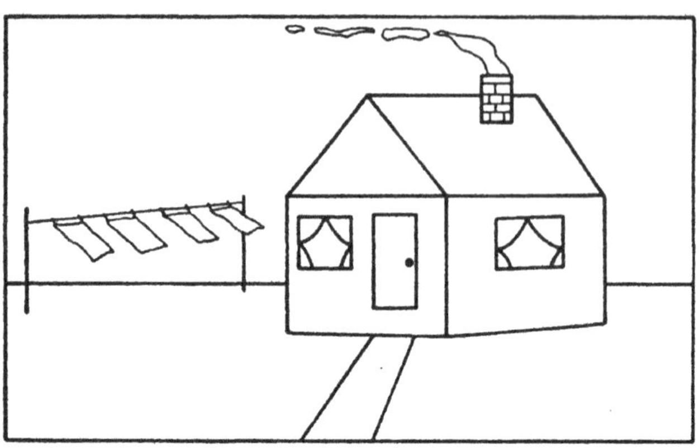

Fig. 4. A sample item from the test Unusual Details. What two things are wrong with this picture?

familiar objects to unusual uses. In this way the items present redefinitions to be evaluated.

A factor known first as "sensitivity to problems" has become recognized as an evaluative ability having to do with implications. One test of the factor, the Apparatus Test, asks for two needed improvements with respect to each of several common devices, such as the telephone or the toaster. The Social Institutions Test, a measure of the same factor, asks what things are wrong with each of several institutions, such as tipping or national elections. We may say that defects or deficiencies are implications of an evaluative kind. Another interpretation would be that seeing defects and deficiencies are evaluations of implications to the effect that the various aspects of something are all right.[4]

## *Some Implications of the Structure of Intellect*

### *For Psychological Theory*

Although factor analysis as generally employed is best designed to investigate ways in which individuals differ from one another, in other words, to discover traits, the results also tell us much about how individuals are alike. Consequently, information regarding the factors and their interrelationships gives us understanding of functioning individuals. The five kinds of intellectual abilities in terms of operations may be said to represent five ways of functioning. The kinds of intellectual abilities distinguished according to varieties of test content and the kinds of abilities distinguished according to varieties of products suggest a classification of basic forms of information or knowledge. The kind of organism suggested by this way of looking at intellect is

4. For further details concerning the intellectual factors, illustrative tests, and the place of the factors in the structure of intellect, see Guilford (1959).

that of an agency for dealing with information of various kinds in various ways. The concepts provided by the distinctions among the intellectual abilities and by their classifications may be very useful in our future investigations of learning, memory, problem solving, invention, and decision making, by whatever method we choose to approach those problems.

*For Vocational Testing*

With about 50 intellectual factors already known, we may say that there are at least 50 ways of being intelligent. It has been facetiously suggested that there seem to be a great many more ways of being stupid, unfortunately. The structure of intellect is a theoretical model that predicts as many as 120 distinct abilities, if every cell of the model contains a factor. Already we know that two cells contain two or more factors each, and there probably are actually other cells of this type. Since the model was first conceived, 12 factors predicted by it have found places in it. There is consequently hope of filling many of the other vacancies, and we may eventually end up with more than 120 abilities.

The major implication for the assessment of intelligence is that to know an individual's intellectual resources thoroughly we shall need a surprisingly large number of scores. It is expected that many of the factors are intercorrelated, so there is some possibility that by appropriate sampling we shall be able to cover the important abilities with a more limited number of tests. At any rate, a multiple-score approach to the assessment of intelligence is definitely indicated in connection with future vocational operations.

Considering the kinds of abilities classified as to content, we may speak roughly of four kinds of intelligence. The abilities involving the use of figural information may be regarded as "concrete" intelligence. The people who depend most upon these abilities deal with concrete things and their properties. Among these people are mechanics, operators of machines, engineers (in some aspects of their work), artists, and musicians.

In the abilities pertaining to symbolic and semantic content, we have two kinds of "abstract" intelligence. Symbolic abilities should be important in learning to recognize words, to spell, and to operate with numbers. Language and mathematics should depend very much upon them, except that in mathematics some aspects, such as geometry, have strong figural involvement. Semantic intelligence is important for understanding things in terms of verbal concepts and hence is important in all courses where the learning of facts and ideas is essential.

In the hypothesized behavioral column of the structure of intellect, which may be roughly described as "social" intelligence, we have some of the most interesting possibilities. Understanding the behavior of others and of ourselves is largely nonverbal in character. The theory suggests as many as 30 abilities in this area, some having to do with understanding, some with productive thinking about behavior, and some with the evaluation of behavior. The theory also suggests that information regarding behavior is also in the form of the six kinds of products that apply elsewhere in the structure of intellect, including units, relations, systems, and so on. The abilities in the area of social intelligence, whatever they prove to be, will possess considerable importance in connection with all those individuals who deal most with other people: teachers, law officials, social workers, therapists, politicians, statesmen, and leaders of other kinds.

### *For Education*

The implications for education are numerous, and I have time just to mention a very few. The most fundamental implication is that we might well undergo transformations with respect to our conception of the learner and of the process of learning. Under the prevailing conception, the learner is a kind of stimulus-response device, much on the order of a vending machine. You put in a coin, and something comes out. The machine learns what reaction to put out when a certain coin is put in. If, instead, we think of the learner as an agent for dealing with information, where information is defined very broadly, we have something more analogous to an electronic computer. We feed a computer information; it stores that information; it uses that information for generating new information, either by way of divergent or convergent thinking; and it evaluates its own results. Advantages that a human learner has over a computer include the step of seeking and discovering new information from sources outside itself and the step of programing itself. Perhaps even these steps will be added to computers, if this has not already been done in some cases.

At any rate, this conception of the learner leads us to the idea that learning is discovery of information, not merely the formation of associations, particularly associations in the form of stimulus-response connections. I am aware of the fact that my proposal is rank heresy. But if we are to make significant progress in our understanding of human learning and particularly our understanding of the so-called higher mental processes of thinking, problem solving, and creative thinking, some drastic modifications are due in our theory.

The idea that education is a matter of training the mind or of training the intellect has been rather unpopular, wherever the prevailing psychological doctrines have been followed. In theory, at least, the emphasis has been upon the learning of rather specific habits or skills. If we take our cue from factor theory, however, we recognize that most learning probably has both specific and general aspects or components. The general aspects may be along the lines of the factors of intellect. This is not to say that the individual's status in each factor is entirely determined by learning. We do not know to what extent each factor is determined by heredity and to what extent by learning. The best position for educators to take is that possibly every intellectual factor can be developed in individuals at least to some extent by learning.

If education has the general objective of developing the intellects of students, it can be suggested that each intellectual factor provides a particular goal at which to aim. Defined by a certain combination of content, operation, and product, each goal ability then calls for certain kinds of practice in order to achieve improvement in it. This implies choice of curriculum and the choice or invention of teaching methods that will most likely accomplish the desired results.

Considering the very great variety of abilities revealed by the factorial exploration of intellect, we are in a better position to ask whether any general intellectual skills are now being neglected in education and whether appropriate balances are being observed. It is often observed these days that we have fallen down in the way of producing resourceful, creative graduates. How true this is, in comparison with other times, I do not know. Perhaps the deficit is noticed because the demands for inventiveness are so much greater at this time. At any rate, realizing that the more conspicuously creative abilities appear to be concentrated in the divergent-thinking category, and also to some extent in the transformation category, we now ask whether we have been giving these skills appropriate exercise. It is probable that we need a better balance of training in the divergent-thinking area as compared with training in convergent thinking and in critical thinking or evaluation.

The structure of intellect as I have presented it to you may or may not stand the test of time. Even if the general form persists, there are likely to be some modifications. Possibly some different kind of model will be invented. Be that as it may, the fact of a multiplicity of intellectual abilities seems well established.

There are many individuals who long for the good old days of simplicity, when we got along with one unanalyzed intelligence. Simplicity certainly has its appeal. But human nature is exceedingly complex, and we may as well face that fact. The rapidly moving events of the world in which we live have forced upon us the need for knowing human intelligence thoroughly. Humanity's peaceful pursuit of happiness depends upon our control of nature and of our own behavior; and this, in turn, depends upon understanding ourselves, including our intellectual resources.

### *References*

Christal, R. E. Factor analytic study of visual memory. *Psychol. Monogr.*, 1958, 72, No. 13 (Whole No. 466).

Guilford, J. P. The structure of intellect. *Psychol. Bull.*, 1956, 53, 267–293.

Guilford, J. P. *Personality*. New York: McGraw-Hill, 1959.

*Dael Wolfle*

# *Diversity of Talent*[1]

A problem of continuing concern is the extent to which we are properly developing and utilizing the nation's intellectual resources. For both realistic and practical reasons it is desirable that we make better provisions than we have in the past for the full development of human talent. The more fundamental reason is that one of the basic ideals of a free society is the provision of opportunity for each person to develop to his full capacity. This ideal has been expressed in many ways, yet from time to time we need to remind ourselves that it lies at the very cornerstone of our form of society. *The Pursuit of Excellence,* the Rockefeller report on education, of which John Gardner (1958) was the principal author, phrased it this way:

> The greatness of a nation may be manifested in many ways —in its purposes, its courage, its moral responsibility, its cultural and scientific eminence, the tenor of its daily life.

1. This paper is based on the Walter Van Dyke Bingham Memorial Lecture given at Columbia University, May 10, 1960. It was first published in the *American Psychologist,* 1960, vol. 15, no. 8 (August), pp. 535–545.

> But ultimately the source of its greatness is in the individuals who constitute the living substance of the nation.
>
> . . . .
>
> Our devotion to a free society can only be understood in terms of these values. It is the only form of society that puts at the very top of its agenda the opportunity of the individual to develop his potentialities. It is the declared enemy of every condition that stunts the intellectual, moral, and spiritual growth of the individual. No society has ever fully succeeded in living up to the stern ideals that a free people set themselves. But only a free society can even address itself to that demanding task.[2]

The idealistic reason for fostering the full development of talent is expressed in the quotation just read. There is also an urgent practical reason: the nation has an increasing need for many kinds of highly developed talent. Earlier in our history, the most critical need was for land for an expanding agriculture and then later for financial capital for an expanding industry. But now the critical need is for men and women with ideas and highly developed talents, men and women who can teach, who can roll back the boundaries of ignorance, who can manage complex organizations, who can perform the diverse and demanding tasks upon which the further development of a free, industrial society depends.

World War II marks the time at which there began to be clear recognition that the need for resources of land and capital had been surpassed by the need for resources of human talent. Prior to World War II we lived through the worst depression in our history. It was not people that we needed, but rather work for

2. From *The Pursuit of Excellence: Education and the Future of America.* Copyright © 1958 by Rockefeller Brothers Fund, Inc. Reprinted by permission of Doubleday & Company, Inc.

the people we had. In the years before the depression, most of the labor force was engaged in farming and in those trades and vocations that make relatively little demand upon man's higher intellectual capacities. It was in World War II that we were pinched for men and brains. It was then that we also began to recognize that invention could be deliberately planned. The scientific and engineering achievements of the war period provided dramatic evidence that some major problems could be solved and some major new inventions produced when imaginative and talented men set their minds to the task. With this wartime demonstration as a model, it seemed likely that organized research could be fruitfully applied on a large scale to industrial problems. There followed a great growth in industrial research, in industrial production, and in interest in the nation's supply of intellectual resources.

My personal involvement in the study of the nation's intellectual resources began in 1950 when I became Director of the Commission on Human Resources and Advanced Training. This commission was established by the American Council of Learned Societies, the American Council on Education, the National Academy of Sciences, and the Social Science Research Council. When the commission's report was published (Wolfle, 1954), it brought together a considerable range of information concerning the supply of talented persons in the United States, the demand for their talents, and the potential supply from which we might draw in the future. Since 1954, public interest in the problem of making fuller use of our intellectual resources has been increased by other studies, by the technological achievements of the USSR, and by a growing recognition of our obligation to help less fortunate nations climb to a higher level of industrial, educational, and personal well-being.

One of the studies of the Commission on Human Resources and Advanced Training dealt with the extent to which the United

States succeeds in educating those young persons who have the intellectual capacity for higher education. Our statistics on this point have been widely used. But the figures we published in 1954 are now out of date and should be replaced. I am glad, therefore, to have the permission of Donald S. Bridgman to quote more recent figures which he has compiled and which will soon be published by the National Science Foundation.

Bridgman was one of my colleagues on the Commission on Human Resources and Advanced Training. He has continued to be interested in how many bright students we are getting, or failing to get, into college. He has considered—as have others—that students in the top 30% of the ability distribution are qualified for college work. Of young men in this ability range, Bridgman's figures show that approximately 45% now graduate from college. Of the 55% who do not, approximately one-fifth fail to finish high school, two-fifths finish high school but do not enter college, and two-fifths enter college but do not finish. Thus we are getting into college about two-thirds of the upper 30% of boys, and about two-thirds of those who enter stay to graduate.

The figures for girls show fewer completing college and more dropping out at earlier stages. Of 100 girls in the top 30% in ability, approximately 30 graduate from college. Of the 70 who do not, about 10 fail to finish high school, 40 finish high school but do not enter college, and 20 enter college but do not graduate.

Of the top 30% in general intellectual ability, for the two sexes combined, nearly 60% enter college, and close to 40% earn bachelor's or higher degrees. If we examine a smaller and more highly selected group, say the top 10% or the top 5% on the intelligence distribution, the retention rates are appreciably higher.

How should we judge these figures? If we compare them with figures from other countries, we have a right to be proud of our record. If we compare them with our own performance in earlier years, we can take pride in the improvement. But if we examine them in terms of our growing need for persons with high ability and advanced education, the current figures give us reason for concern. We should seek to increase the percentage of able young men and women who receive a higher education, but even as we seek that increase we can already foresee the limits on future improvement under our present methods of selection and education. As we look to the future, we must consider how to make better use of our resources of talent.

### *The Encouragement of Talent*

The obvious first response to this problem is that we should be more active in the encouragement of talented young persons. Thus Charles H. Brower (1960), President of the advertising firm Batten, Barton, Durstine, and Osborne, said recently to the Advertising Federation of America:

> I ask only that we look for talent and excellence as avidly as we look for . . . many of our less valuable natural resources.
> . . . .
> Our educators, our ministers, our editors, our businessmen, our unions, and our organizations . . . should join in a mammoth talent hunt to uncover [the] treasure of brains which . . . is hiding in unlikely places all over America.

In actuality, a talent hunt has long characterized both the American culture and a number of other cultures. Part of this hunt has been systematically organized; much of it has been informal, unorganized, and on an individual basis.

Walter Bingham once told me that he approached the end of high school with no thought of entering college. One day one of his teachers took him aside and planted the idea that led him to enroll at Kansas University the following fall. I wonder how often a similar scene has occurred in the early lives of men and women who later entered the professional or learned fields. George Beadle, who was awarded the 1958 Nobel Prize in Physiology and Medicine, tells an almost identical story: a Nebraska farm boyhood, a father uninterested in higher education, and an inspiring teacher who urged the future Nobel laureate to enter the University of Nebraska. There must be many other eminent men and women who could tell similar stories: bright, industrious students with potentialities far exceeding the range of vision acquired from home and community, whose sights were lifted by a teacher or an older friend who took the trouble to encourage talent. I am glad that Bingham told me how he was encouraged to go to college, for perhaps that experience helps to explain his abiding interest in the identification and encouragement of talented youngsters.

The incident also illustrates the principle to which I wish to give first attention. The principle is this: talent requires encouragement. Certainly there are exceptions, or at least apparent exceptions: each of us could name greatly gifted men who rose from poor surroundings, overcoming great obstacles, seemingly driven by a force that no hardships and no obstacles could impede. There may be exceptions, but it is neither safe nor realistic to assume that high ability is always accompanied by high motivation, that human talent will override obstacles to find its own way to fruition. Nor is it safe to assume that the necessary inspiration or encouragement will always be provided by the family.

In an illuminating study of the role of personal encouragement in the lives of bright students, Swanson (1955) interviewed men who, some twenty years earlier, had been superior high school seniors. Some of these men had gone to college; others had quit at the end of high school. Swanson tried to find out what influences had determined which of these men had gone to college and which had not. One of the clearest differences was the simple fact that someone—a teacher, a minister, a relative, or a friend—had encouraged some of the men to go to college, while others could not recall that anyone had ever suggested that they should continue formal education beyond high school. Certainly other factors than this one were involved; much besides a few conversations on the topic determines how long a student stays in school. But it is significant that the men who went to college were usually actively encouraged to do so, sometimes encouraged by several people, while those who did not enter college could not recall this kind of personal encouragement.

Walter Bingham might or might not have attended college had his teacher not encouraged him. I think perhaps he might, for another story of his youth shows a character already marked by determination and self-confidence. He made straight A's his first year in college, a good record for a 16-year-old boy who was the youngest student on the campus. But he established no firm friendships and did not want to return to Kansas University. Where should he go? He applied to two colleges, he told me. One promptly accepted him; the other did not reply. When summer came to an end and it was again time to go off to college, in which direction should he head: to the college that had accepted him or to the one that had ignored him? The safe and cautious solution would have been to go to the college that had accepted him, but young Walter was more venturesome. He concluded that the college that was eager to have him must not have many good students and that the college that did not seem to care whether he came or not must therefore be the better institution. So, off he went to Beloit, the college that had not acknowledged his application, but that did accept him on arrival and that turned his interest toward psychology. I suspect that a 17-year-old boy who possessed the self-assurance evident in this decision might well have gone to college anyway, whether or not a particular teacher had urged him. But we cannot be sure. Perhaps we are able to honor Bingham because we are in reality also honoring the high school teacher who recognized his talent and encouraged him to develop it.

Anecdotes are useful if they illustrate a significant principle, but it is time to return to the principle: talent requires encouragement if it is to reach its full development. The encouragement may come from parents or other interested individuals, or encouragement may be built into the customs and traditions that characterize a particular social group. Scotland has produced an unusually large number of notable men. This high intellectual productivity has been explained as resulting from widespread interest among the Scots in seeking out and encouraging talent. Whether this explanation would withstand critical analysis, I do not know, but that there are major differences in intellectual productivity among different social and ethnic groups is completely clear.

### *Social Factors in Talent Development*

About ten years ago the Social Science Research Council's Committee on the Identification of Talent began an investigation of some of these differences. The committee received a substantial grant from the John and Mary R. Markle Foundation and decided that this grant should not be used in attempts to improve aptitude tests or other existing methods of identifying talent, but should rather be used to investigate some of the social conditions that help to determine how talent manifests itself and how it is stunted or made to blossom. One of the studies that we supported was by Fred Strodtbeck (1958). Strodtbeck started by selecting a number of bright, teen-age boys. Half were Jewish, half Italian. He then set out to analyze the Italian-Jewish cultural differences and to determine how these differences influence the aspirations and education of growing boys. This he did by studying the values that characterized the thinking of the families of each of his subjects, and the patterns of social interaction among the father, the mother, and the bright son. He found that in a number of quite detailed respects Jews have values more likely to promote high achievement than do Italians and that there is greater agreement among Jewish family members on these values.

I do not want to go into detail concerning Strodtbeck's study, but I cite it as an example of the possibility of investigating the social factors that influence the extent to which potentially high ability will actually be developed. I might have cited other studies, such as the Quincy (Illinois) Youth Development Project of Robert F. De Haan and Robert J. Havighurst, or the different approach of Anne Roe, or the still different works of Samuel Stouffer. Instead of extending this list, let me merely call attention to the importance of learning more than we now know about the social conditions that influence the development and utilization of talent. We need better information concerning the family as a social system, the school as a social system, and the ways in which these social systems encourage talent or hinder its development.

### *Policy for Talent Development*

The encouragement of talent is clearly desirable, and so is the better understanding of the social conditions that aid or hinder its development, both because the individual with talent is thus more likely to reach closer to his full potential and because the nation is more likely to gain the advantage of his high ability. But it is not sufficient simply to say that we should encourage talent wherever we find it. There is an additional, and psychologically more interesting, question to take up.

This psychologically more interesting question has to do with the development of an underlying policy or strategy of talent development. If one of us were suddenly assigned responsibility for developing a national policy of talent development, I wonder what he would do. No single one of us is likely to be given this responsibility, but collectively it is shared by many persons, whether they realize it or not. Every person who constructs or interprets a test or other measure for the selection of scholarship or fellowship winners, every college admissions officer, every guidance counselor, every educational philosopher or administrator, and every teacher daily makes decisions that in fact do help to determine how the nation's intellectual resources are developed and utilized. Their actions constitute our unanalyzed, but nonetheless determining, present policy.

We have, in the past, concerned ourselves chiefly with the techniques of identifying talented persons and furthering their education. So long as our work is controlled primarily by techniques, the major directions will be determined by the techniques themselves, the criteria that we find most reliable, and relevant statistical and experimental considerations. These factors should continue to concern us. But by themselves they are not enough. It is time to give consideration to questions of social value, purpose, or ultimate objective. I suggest that it is time for those of us who are professionally most concerned to consider the policy issues and to try to develop a strategy that will maximize the achievement and social value of the persons whose talents we seek to identify and develop.

Two aspects of such a policy are obvious. First is the desirability of encouraging the full development of all forms of socially useful talent. Of this point I have already spoken. Second is the need for a better understanding of the social and cultural factors that stimulate or retard the development of talent. Of the need for research I have also spoken.

After these two points, what comes next? In addition to identifying talented youngsters and helping them to secure an education commensurate with their abilities, in addition to conducting research, we must also consider how the talent we are developing can be so distributed as to result in the greatest accomplishment. The recommendation that I will make on this point is likely to be controversial. In order to point up the issue clearly, I will start with what may seem to be an extreme point of view.

### *The Value of Diversity*

In the selection and education of persons of ability, it is advantageous to a society to seek the greatest achievable diversity of talent: diversity within an individual, among the members of an occupational group, and among the individuals who constitute a society.

In speaking of diversity among individuals, I am using words in their ordinary meaning; but when I speak of diversity within an individual, the expression sounds strange. There is no customary term for the idea I am trying to express, for the adjectives with good connotations mean the opposite of what I am trying to say. I am not talking about the well-rounded individual, or the broad scholar, or the man of many talents. These are qualities we ordinarily respect; but I wish to make a case for the opposite, for the man who has developed some of his talents so highly that he cannot be well-rounded, for the one who may be called uneven or one-sided but in whom at least one side has been developed to the level of real superiority. For the sake of symmetry with the concept of diversity among individuals, I have called this kind of development diversity within an individual. If the expression still seems strange, its meaning will become clearer as we go along.

One further explanation is essential. I do not wish to maximize variance or diversity by having some persons very bright and others very dull. Obviously we want each person to reach the highest level of which he is capable. But even if we were doing as well as we know how to do in the identification and education of talented persons, the problem of optimal deployment of their various talents would still be a question of undiminished psychological and social interest. Even under these circumstances, a strong case can be made for the proposition that the value of a nation's intellectual resources—or the total achievement—would be maximized by maximizing the variety of abilities within and among individuals. This is not a new idea; but the point needs repetition and also needs analysis, for even though we agree upon the value of diversity, strong forces are constantly at work in the opposite direction. These forces tend to make us more, rather than less, alike and tend to prevent the uneven development of a talented individual.

Many of the methods that have been developed for dealing with people in groups have the effect of reducing the variability among the group members. Examples are the use of uniform lesson assignments and the use of general aptitude measures and the average grade or the rank in class as devices for selecting students for the next higher educational level. Advertising procedures, trade union policies, wage scales, and a variety of other forces also work in the direction of uniformity rather than diversity. These tendencies are supported by popular attitudes that place a premium on uniformity and conformity rather than upon diversity and individuality. Lyle Spencer quotes the mother of three bright children as saying: "I'm not interested in geniuses, all I want to do is to raise my kids to be normal, well-adjusted adults." Many parents would agree; they want their children to be like other children, and not to be different. Teachers, too, sometimes express this attitude. De Haan and Havighurst (1957) quote a teacher as saying: "When I am finished with my class in June, the slow children are a little faster, and the fast have slowed down a bit."

Years ago, Truman Kelley protested this attitude and leveled his guns against school teachers and officials who exhibit it. He called them pedagogical plainsmen and accused them of preferring intellectual plains to intellectual hills and valleys. They were, he wrote, so obsessed with averages and norms that they devoted themselves to "the weary process of shovelling to fill valleys and steady erosion to remove mountains of human capacity."

Had Harold Benjamin not already pre-empted the title, I might have called this address "The Cultivation of Idiosyncrasy," for the major point of my argument is that the cultivation of diversity is desirable both for the individual young persons whose futures lie in our hands and for the society in which they will live and work. I cannot use Benjamin's title, but I can quote a few of his paragraphs (1955). The wit and humor with which he approached serious problems has illuminated many an educational discussion, and the fable he used in opening the Inglis lecture at Harvard in 1949 illustrates the point I want to make. The fable is the story of the school in the woods.

> All the animals had to take all the subjects. Swimming, running, jumping, climbing, and flying made up the required curriculum.
>
> . . . .
>
> Some animals, of course, were better students than others. The squirrel, for example, got straight A's from the first in running, jumping, and climbing. He got a good passing grade, moreover, in swimming. It looked as though he would make Phi Beta Kappa in his junior year, but he had trouble with flying. Not that he was unable to fly. He could fly. He

> climbed to the top of tree after tree and sailed through the air to neighboring trees with ease. As he modestly observed, he was a flying squirrel by race. The teacher of flying pointed out, however, that the squirrel was always losing altitude in his gliding and insisted that he should take off in the approved fashion from the ground. Indeed, the teacher decided that the taking-off-from-the-ground unit had to be mastered first, as was logical, and so he drilled the squirrel day after day on the take-off.
>
> . . . .
>
> The squirrel tried hard. He tried so hard he got severe Charley horses in both hind legs, and thus crippled he became incapable even of running, jumping, or climbing. He left school a failure, and died soon thereafter of starvation, being unable to gather and store nuts.

Benjamin continued the fable to relate the difficulties of the snake, the eagle, and the gopher. I shall quote only the story of the eagle.

> The eagle was a truly brilliant student. His flying was superb, his running and jumping were of the best, and he even passed the swimming test, although the teacher tried to keep him from using his wings too much. By employing his talons and beak, moreover, he could climb after a fashion and no doubt he would have been able to pass that course, too, except that he always flew to the top of the problem tree or cliff when the teacher's back was turned and sat there lazily in the sun, preening his feathers and staring arrogantly down at his fellow students climbing up the hard way. The teachers reasoned with him to no avail. He would not study climbing seriously. At first he turned aside the faculty's importunities with relatively mild wisecracks and innuendoes, but as the teachers put more pressure upon him he reacted

> with more and more feeling . . . [and finally quit school altogether].

I wonder how many human students have been similarly frustrated and had their talents stunted by being required to climb slowly step by step, instead of being encouraged to soar rapidly to the heights of which they were capable.

I have said that it is socially valuable to maximize diversity. Now let me try to prove the point. I should like to be able to give a rigorous proof; for, if the assertion is correct, there flow from it a number of implications for the professional work of psychologists, guidance counselors, teachers, and all who deal professionally with the identification, education, and utilization of talented persons. The proof cannot be rigorous, for we do not have adequate measures of amount of talent, of achievement, or of the social value of achievement. But it is possible to analyze these variables and to examine their interrelationships. The exercise leads convincingly to the conclusion that maximum diversity results in maximum social value.

Let us start the analysis with two points on which there is general agreement. The first is that individuals vary in the total amount of talent or ability they possess. This simple statement overlooks the whole nature-nurture problem, the effects of education, and all of the difficulties of measuring talent. Moreover, it oversimplifies the whole matter by treating ability as a trait that an individual possesses rather than as an attribute of the behavior he exhibits. Nevertheless, to say that different individuals possess different total amounts of ability is a convenient way of stating an idea that is generally accepted.

The second point is that ability is not a unitary trait but expresses itself in various forms or special abilities. We may side with L. L. Thurstone in believing that a relatively small number of more or less independent primary abilities provide a satisfactory description of human ability, or we may side with Godfrey Thompson in postulating a large number of highly specialized abilities. For our purpose, it makes little difference which of these positions one prefers. All that is essential is that we agree that ability is a many-sided affair and that an individual may be better in one kind of ability than he is in another.

Now let us suppose that an individual could distribute his ability over various kinds of performances in any way he preferred. Within limits, this is a reasonable proposition, for each individual does exercise some control. If a student neglects the academic subjects in order to practice on the piano, he will become a better pianist, and a poorer scholar. Alternatively, he can concentrate on something else and neglect the piano entirely. Students constantly make educational decisions, allocate study time, choose schools, select reading matter, or neglect their studies. All such decisions influence the extent to which one or another ability will be developed.

Now let us move from this realistic situation to its unrealistic limit, and to simplify the task let us arbitrarily assign some numbers to the situation. Suppose that a given individual has 1,000 units of ability—another individual might have more or fewer—and let us suppose that he can distribute these 1,000 units in any way he chooses over 20 different kinds of ability. If he wishes to be a completely well-rounded individual, he would assign 50 units to each of the 20 abilities. Or, he might elect the 10 kinds of ability that he thinks most important and assign 100 units to each, neglecting completely the other 10 kinds of ability because they seem to him to be unimportant. Or, at the extreme, as a kind of talent gambler, he might stake his whole 1,000 units on one kind of ability and neglect the other 19 completely. Which of these ways of distributing his total talent fund would be best for the individual?

A parallel question can be asked from the point of view of

society. Suppose that society rather than the individual decides how the 1,000 units will be distributed. Which would best serve society: to assign 50 units to each of 20 different kinds of ability, 100 units to each of 10 kinds, or the whole 1,000 units to a single ability?

We cannot answer these questions without considering the values involved. In real life, these values are often conflicting. The eminent young mathematician has to help care for the children, occasionally to repair the lawn mower, and take his turn in helping to run the affairs of the local Boy Scout troop. As a mathematician, he might like to concentrate all of his units of ability on mathematics. But as a human being with other interests, he has to save some of those units for other and quite nonmathematical kinds of ability and achievement. In real life, many conflicting value considerations are involved, but let us neglect them for the time being and concentrate on the problem of maximizing the social value of human talents.

The value that society places upon different levels of accomplishment does not vary directly with the amount of achievement or its underlying ability, but increases more rapidly than does the amount. A graph relating amount of talent and its social value would be a curve rather than a straight line—doubling the amount of ability more than doubles its value; doubling again the amount again more than doubles the value. The relationship can be illustrated with some arbitrary numbers: if one unit of ability is worth one dollar to society, 50 units are worth more than $50; perhaps 50 units are worth $100. Similarly for larger amounts, 100 units may be worth $500, and 1,000 units may be so valuable as to be priceless. These particular numbers are arbitrary, but that the relationship is nonlinear is clear. The salaries paid to chemists or engineers or members of other professions are not symmetrically distributed about a mean. The distributions are skewed, with a longer tail above the mean than below it. Moreover, there is general recognition that the salaries paid to the ablest people fall far short of being commensurate with their ability. On the ordinary scale of salaries for writers, physicists, and public servants, we make no effort to pay appropriate salaries to a Shakespeare, an Einstein, or a Winston Churchill.

We use other means to compensate outstanding persons whose salaries are not commensurate with their ability. We award Gold Medals to Olympic winners, Nobel Prizes to great scientists, Pulitzer Prizes to outstanding authors and editors, and we have other honors with which we recognize excellence in other fields. Partly by the amounts of money paid for different levels of ability and partly in other forms of compensation, society demonstrates that the value it places on talent increases more rapidly than does the amount of talent.

Now we can return to the question of the most valuable way of distributing talents. From the standpoint of society, the best way to distribute talent is to take maximum advantage of differences in aptitude, interest, and motivation by having each individual concentrate on the thing he can do best. Instead of having the 1,000-unit man distribute his ability 50 units on each of 20 kinds of ability or 100 units on each of 10, have him concentrate the whole 1,000 units on a single ability. In Harold Benjamin's fable, have the eagle be the best flyer in the world and forget about his ability to swim or climb, have the squirrel be the best climber in the world and stop worrying about his inability to fly. In human affairs, follow the same principle. Have one man be the best he can possibly become in one line and another the best he can possibly become in another line. Thus we would have the best physicist, the best poet, the best mathematician, and the best dramatist possible. The total value of the talents so distributed would be incomparably greater than would be the value of the same number of units of talent spread more uniformly over the different men and the different abilities involved.

Recommending that each person be helped to achieve the highest level he can reach in the area in which he has the greatest talent and interest is not the same as recommending that every scholar be a narrow specialist. Some, however, should be specialists, and some should specialize in relatively narrow fields. Physics is generally recognized as the most highly developed science. Further advances are most likely to be made by physicists who concentrate on a particular area of physics. Thus we want highly specialized physicists. But we also want physicists of wider interest and knowledge: persons who can bridge the gaps between physics and biology or physics and other sciences, persons who are interested in the practical applications of physical principles, and persons who are interested in attempting to translate physics into terms that the rest of us can try to understand. This diversity among physicists is essential if physics itself is to advance and if other fields of intellectual and practical endeavor are to benefit maximally from those advances.

From the standpoint of social value, maximum diversity would be the ideal; but like many another ideal, it is unattainable. In real life we must recognize that the best mathematician in the world must do something besides mathematics and that the best poet cannot spend all his energy on poetry. But the fact that the extreme case is unrealistic does not destroy the principle. The principle is this, and I state it now in realistic rather than imaginary terms: to the extent that we can control the distribution of talent, it is socially desirable to maximize the diversity, both within and among individuals.

This is the ideal. Before we consider methods of reaching toward that ideal, it is worthwhile briefly to look at its opposite, for then we will have set the boundaries within which we can maneuver in our educational and guidance practices.

In *Brave New World,* Aldous Huxley (1932) described a society in which most individuals were born as members of batches. Born, you will remember, is not the right word: old-fashioned human birth had been replaced by a kind of controlled embryology in which any desired number of identical individuals could be developed from a single fertilized egg. The eggs were developed in vitro, and at the proper time babies, instead of being born, were decanted. Through controlled nutrition, and through proper training and education, the members of a batch could be made to have any desired level of ability, and all the members of a batch were as alike as identical twins that had been reared together. We can dismiss *Brave New World* as satirical exaggeration; but we cannot dismiss the kind of society that Huxley was satirizing, for there are forces in society that tend in the direction of homogeneity, and there are cultural values that make homogeneity seem desirable.

Between the unreality of *Brave New World* and the unreality of maximum diversity there is a wide range. Within this range we have considerable room to choose the kind of society we want ours to be. Ultimately the essential choices will be made by the nation as a whole, through the processes of democratic action. But in a more immediate sense, and on the important aspect of talent distribution, choices must be made by those persons who are professionally engaged in the development and handling of talent.

As to how far we should go in the direction of diversity, I have only two suggestions, and both must be stated in general terms. One is that we should go as far as we can. The other is that the greater the ability with which we are dealing, the greater is the amount of idiosyncrasy we can tolerate. The brief and brilliant career of the Indian mathematician Ramanujan (Newman, 1957) illustrates both principles. The name may be strange, for Ramanujan was a mathematicians' mathematician and was little known outside of mathematical circles. Yet he has been described as "quite the most extraordinary mathematician of our time." At the age of 15, he was loaned a copy of Carr's *Synopsis of Pure*

*Mathematics.* This was all he had, and all he needed, to start him off on a strange, unorthodox, and inspired career of mathematical innovation. Working completely alone, he rediscovered much that had been developed by earlier mathematicians; he followed some false leads and made some mistakes; but in some fields of mathematics his power and originality went beyond any other mathematician in the world.

On the basis of his obvious brilliance, he was given a scholarship; but he lost it at the end of the first term because he failed his examination in English. He never did earn a university degree; but at the age of 25, after working for some years as a clerk, he was given a fellowship at Cambridge where he went to work with G. H. Hardy. Hardy faced the problem of deciding how much he should let Ramanujan go his own way, and how much he should try to correct his mistakes and make him into a more orthodox mathematician. Hardy expressed his dilemma in these words:

> It was impossible to ask such a man to submit to systematic instruction, to try to learn mathematics from the beginning once more. I was afraid too that, if I insisted unduly on matters which Ramanujan found irksome, I might destroy his confidence or break the spell of his inspiration. On the other hand there were things of which it was impossible that he should remain in ignorance. . . . It was impossible to let him go through life supposing that all the zeros of the Zeta-function were real.

The moral of the story is that, if we are dealing with a Ramanujan, we can put up with a great deal of eccentricity; if we are dealing with a lesser mind, we can insist on more conformity. Even with a Ramanujan there is a limit, but let us in all cases push that limit as far out as we can.

### *Implications*

Let me now briefly suggest some of the implications of the principle that it is socially valuable to increase the diversity of talent. Each of these implications relates to practices that are under our professional control.

The first implication is that it is desirable to make wider use of tests of special ability or aptitude to supplement our tests of general ability. De Haan and Havighurst (1957) found, in a survey of 40 school systems, that nearly all used tests of general intellectual ability as a means of appraising the potential of their students, but only 3 used tests of special aptitudes. Failure to use special tests increases the danger of overlooking students with unusually high potential in art, music, creative writing, and other abilities that are not well measured by the usual tests of general intellectual aptitude.

A second implication is that it is desirable to increase the use of separate scores for separate types of ability and to decrease the use of single scores that represent the sum or combination of several part scores. When students are being selected for awards or for admission to the next higher educational level, global measures are the easiest ones to use. Moreover, global measures are the ones that are likely to give the highest validity coefficients. Most of our usual measures of success are factorially complex and can be better predicted by factorially complex tests than by factorially simpler ones.

We pay a price, however, for the ease of use and for the higher validity of general measures of aptitude. The price we pay for using general measures is that we reduce the apparent size of the pool of talent on which we can draw. Relying solely on tests of general intellectual aptitude reduces the size of the talent pool because various kinds of ability, although usually positively correlated with one another, are by no means perfectly correlated.

In the Quincy youth development study, selection of the top 10% of the children in general intellectual ability, the top 10% in leadership, and the top 2% in drawing ability included 16% of the total population. The authors estimate that, had they also included the top 10% each in music, dramatic ability, creative writing, and mechanical ability, they would have brought into their talent development program 20–25% of the total child population (De Haan & Havighurst, 1957).

In Kenneth Little's study (1958) of Wisconsin high school graduates, he used the usual measures of high school grades and general intelligence. But he went beyond these measures by asking the teachers to identify those of their students who were specially gifted in any field. About 20% of the students so identified had not ranked in the upper quarter of their graduating class in either general scholastic achievement or general mental ability. Included were students whom the teachers identified as being specially gifted in art, music, science, and other fields. Clearly the use of tests of special aptitude and the use of individual grades and scores rather than averages identifies a larger number of talented young persons and thus lays the basis for the development of a larger and more diversified talent pool.

An opportunity to use the more detailed information made available by separate scores is found in the award of scholarships and fellowships. The person who is high on every score and thus high on the sum or average of his scores should, of course, be encouraged to continue his education, and such students clearly merit awards, scholarships, and fellowships. But when we drop down a step or two below the generally superior level, we still tend to base awards on the average score instead of looking for evidence of exceptionally high merit in individual fields or abilities. I would suggest that in awarding scholarships when we reach this slightly lower general level, we make some of the awards to students who have earned very high marks on individual tests or measures of ability. We will probably experience some lowering of validity coefficients, we may make awards to a few unproductive eccentrics; but we will enhance our chances of picking up a few persons so highly gifted and so intensely interested along one line that they have neglected, or rebelliously disdained, to keep pace with their fellows in other lines.

A third implication is that the patterning of abilities should be avoided in the selection or guidance of persons entering or contemplating entering a particular occupation. You may recall the long history of unsuccessful efforts to find the optimal pattern of abilities and personality traits that characterize the successful members of an occupational group. No one has stated the hope for such patterns better than Clark Hull (1928) who, thirty years ago, pointed out that vocational guidance would be easy if we had measures of the various kinds of ability and if we had carried out the analyses necessary to determine the weight with which each type of ability enters into the determination of success in each of a variety of occupations. Under the system that Hull anticipated, an applicant for vocational guidance would be given a battery of tests that measured all of the major types of ability. His scores on these tests would be fed into a computer which already contained in its storage unit the regression weights of each ability on each of a variety of occupations. The sum of the products of the ability scores and the corresponding regression weights for a given occupation would then be automatically computed and would represent the applicant's predicted standard score for success in that occupation. With a modern computer, it would be possible to determine very quickly the predicted standard scores for success in each of a large number of occupations.

In the days since Hull wrote this description, the necessary computers have reached a high stage of development; tests of different kinds of ability have been improved, although not nearly so much as the computers. But we have also learned enough about ability, vocations, and the factors that make for success to have concluded that the kind of differential prediction that Hull described is not feasible. A major reason is that relatively diverse patterns of ability are consistent with success in a single vocation. Any professional field includes opportunities for such a variety of persons—persons differing in abilities and differing in personality traits—that there is no simple or single pattern that is either essential or sufficient. Consider engineering, or medicine, or psychology, or any other field of work that demands intellectual ability. Each title covers a wide variety of tasks; each field includes opportunities for a wide variety of persons.

The search for a pattern characteristic of each profession has failed. As I have considered this failure, I have become convinced that we were on the wrong track in looking for distinctive patterns. For law, medicine, engineering, psychology, and other fields are enriched by having within their ranks a wide range of patterns of ability.

### *Conclusion*

It would be possible to present other implications of the values of diversity, implications for the guidance and for the education of talented students. A general discussion of these fields would take far too long, and I will refrain, for now it is time to conclude. The needs of the nation for highly developed talent are growing and will continue to grow. This is an inevitable feature of the kind of complex, industrialized, specialized society in which we live. If we are to make full use of our intellectual resources, the first requisite is that we employ all the means at our command to encourage the development of talent. The second requisite is that they learn more about the social factors that aid or impede the development of talent.

I expect that these two points are noncontroversial. I am not so sure about the third point that I have advanced. Some of you may disagree with part or all of what I have said about the strategy of optimal distribution or deployment of talent. I readily grant the privilege of disagreement, for you have given me the opportunity to argue that we should go beyond personal action and beyond scientific research to consider the question of how our professional activities concerned with talent can be supported and unified by an underlying policy of talent development—a policy that seeks to maximize achievement and thus to maximize the value to society of our resources of talent.

What I have attempted to do is to state the first principles of a strategy of talent development, a strategy that provides a unifying rationale for our efforts to improve the construction and interpretation of tests, and the counseling, guidance, and education of talented young minds. The strategy is one of increasing the diversity of talent, in an individual, within an occupation, and in society. There will always be counterpressures that must be respected; but to the extent that we succeed in increasing the diversity of talent, we will have increased its value to society.

### *References*


Benjamin, H. *The cultivation of idiosyncrasy.* Cambridge, Mass.: Harvard Univer. Press, 1955.

Bridgman, D. S. *Losses of intellectual talent from the educational system prior to graduation from college.* Washington, D.C.: NSF.

Brower, C. H. The year of the rat. Address to Advertising Federation of America, Boston, February 9, 1960.

De Haan, R. F., & Havighurst, R. J. *Educating gifted children.* Chicago: Univer. Chicago Press, 1957.

Gardner, J. W., *et al. The pursuit of excellence: education and the future of America.* (The "Rockefeller" report on education.) Garden City, N.Y.: Doubleday, 1958.

Hull, C. L. *Aptitude testing.* Yonkers-on-Hudson, N.Y.: World Book, 1928.

Huxley, A. *Brave new world.* Garden City, N.Y.: Doubleday, Doran, 1932.

Little, J. K. A state-wide inquiry into decisions of youth about education beyond high school. University of Wisconsin, 1958.

Newman, J. R. Srinivasa Ramanujan. In *Lives in science.* New York: Simon & Schuster, 1957, pp. 257–269.

Strodtbeck, F. L. Family interaction, values, and achievement. In D. C. McClelland *et al., Talent and society.* Princeton, N.J.: Van Nostrand, 1958, pp. 135–194.

Swanson, E. O. Is college education worthwhile? *J. counsel. Psychol.,* 1955, 2, 176–181.

Wolfle, D. *America's resources of specialized talent.* New York: Harper, 1954.

*John M. Stalnaker*

# *Recognizing and Encouraging Talent*[1]

The National Merit Scholarship Program was created some 5 years ago as a means of arousing the public's awareness of and respect for intellectual talent and in this way to encourage the development of such talent. Ideally, a scholarship program will extend its influence far beyond the small group of students who are actually given scholarships. By helping to foster a climate of opinion favorable to intellectual excellence, it will stimulate latent talent.

One of the popular themes of the day is the need to develop fully our human resources. There is no need to labor the point here, except to say that this need is the reason for the Merit Program. Suffice it to observe that the saying, "Knowledge is power," has never been more true than it is today, and that knowledge has become so complex and extensive that more and higher education are almost absolute requisites for advancing our knowl-

1. This paper is based on the Walter Van Dyke Bingham Memorial Lecture given at Carnegie Institute of Technology, March 23, 1961. It was first published in the *American Psychologist*, 1961, vol. 16, no. 8 (August), pp. 513–522.

edge—and advance it we must on many fronts. Good minds are required even to keep up with the new developments today. Only the most talented minds will make new breakthroughs for us. Higher education is becoming a requirement, not only for individual fulfillment, but also for national survival in this day when man-made weapons are capable of destroying the world.

Moreover, the untrained and the uneducated have greater and greater difficulty in finding a useful place in the modern world. Whitehead's prophecy that there will be no appeal from the judgment which will be pronounced on the uneducated is about to become true.

As a nation we are slowly awakening to our responsibilities in education. To be sure, we have since our founding shown a certain dedication to universal education. In no major country in the world today is education more widely available than in the United States. There are colleges in every state and in every major city, and the number of these institutions is constantly increasing. Today, over half of our secondary school graduates enter college and the proportion is increasing each year.

But until recently we have not been concerned that our youth learn at as fast a pace as their ability permits the basic principles of those subjects without which life in the modern world is inconceivable. While paying lip service to the ideal of universal education, we have neglected our schools (and their teachers). We have asked that teachers instruct our children without demanding effort from the students. The quality of educational opportunity is poor in many places and the educational standards low. Universal availability of high quality education will provide a proving ground for all youth to show their ability.

Now we are faced with a serious international situation which threatens our very existence. The power which recognizes talent and develops it to the productive stage, quickly and in quantity, has the best chance of winning the race.

When the National Merit Scholarship Corporation was created in mid-1955, Sputnik I was not for another 2 years to arouse the American public to a new concern about the nature and quality of its education. The prevailing atmosphere in the schools at that time was a peaceful calm. Adjustment and contentment were the goals. Schools were permissive, relatively noncompetitive, and paid little attention to standards of performance. There were no priorities in subject matter; courses were offered in homemaking, family living, cooking, and the like. Competition was de-emphasized. Every child should enjoy success. High school graduates were often not able to read or write at the level required for college work. As a result remedial courses were common in the colleges.

While there was much talk about talent, the temper of the people encouraged competition in the sports rather than the academic arena. Little league ball clubs could count on parental interest, financing, and guidance. As Elmo Roper has observed: "We have no folk tradition that seeks out and trains and sponsors and takes pride in exceptional intellectual talent. There are no little leagues of the mind."

What a nation respects and honors tends to prosper and grow. The star player on the winning basketball team can be assured of great public recognition and acclaim. The entire town will turn out to honor him. Newspapers will devote space to his amazing performance. The school itself may dismiss classes to celebrate the great victory. College scouts and "admission counselors" will visit him. Young children notice what is honored by adults, what adults judge to be important.

The serious, able youngster who devoted himself to scholarly work received no such public acclaim back in the days before 1955. His classmates regarded him as a "brain"—a term of opprobrium at that time—and ignored him. No public recognition stimulated him to greater effort. His juniors did not look up to him with envy in their hearts and a determination to follow in his footsteps.

The National Merit Scholarship Program was created to help to change this dismal, distorted picture. Could some of the elements of the contest be brought into the intellectual field? Conant in his *Citadel of Learning* remarked that the spirit of competition need not be deplored; it might under certain conditions be a healthy motivating force in the academic field. "Local enthusiasm," he said, "needs to be aroused for discovering and adequately educating those who are intellectually gifted."

The problem was to design a contest in the intellectual field suitable for students in the upper years of high school. Scholarships would be the incentive—the motive power—and the program would have several important objectives.

First of all, the Merit Program would be a champion of able and talented youth. Most scholarship money is controlled by a relatively small number of colleges, who use it mostly for institutional promotion and development. Much of it is spent attracting the talented student from one college to another. The Merit Program, on the other hand, finds able students, wherever they may be, and helps them attend any college they select and study any curriculum of interest to them.

Another objective of the Merit Program would be to arouse public interest in intellectual talent. With the help of the secondary schools of the nation—all 25,000 of them—the Merit Program launched a dramatic campaign to find and publicize exceptionally able students. The top performers in such a national contest would receive notice in the local press, and thus the townspeople would become aware of that most precious of all their resources, talented local youngsters.

It was hoped that the Merit Program would be a mechanism to assure—to the extent of its resources—that no unusually talented student was denied a college education because of the economic status of his family. In addition to offering a substantial number of scholarships itself, the Merit Program notifies other scholarship agencies about the students it finds, thus helping exceptional students to obtain financial aid.

The Merit Program had as another objective the prevention of wasteful duplication. Any number of sponsors can utilize without cost the selection mechanism of the Merit Program to locate students having the particular characteristics of interest to them, so that they can support such students in their further education.

The Merit Program was aimed to help create a climate of opinion in which intellectual excellence would be respected and encouraged. "The United States has not achieved the tradition of respect for learning in all fields that is so much a part of the culture of other peoples," writes the Director of the National Science Foundation, Alan T. Waterman. "Above all, we must strive for a climate of opinion that will be favorable to our intellectual as well as creative activities."

Perhaps most important of all, the Merit Program, by gathering data on able students throughout the land, will contribute to our knowledge about the location, background, and development of unusual intellectual talent. Research activities constitute an integral and basic part of the Merit Program operation.

These several hoped-for outcomes are broad as well as deep, and they will not be achieved easily or quickly. Many obstacles were anticipated.

Legally, the National Merit Scholarship Corporation is a nonprofit corporation in the State of Illinois. It restricts its activities to scholarship matters but within that field it handles all phases. An independent corporation not responsible to any other organization or group, it is controlled by a board of 22 Directors drawn from the fields of business, higher education, and secondary education. The board creates the basic policies of the corporation and oversees its general operations.

In addition to this board, there is an advisory council which recommends to the corporation's President procedures which will have the greatest educational values. There is also a research advisory board which reviews research activities and recommends new directions for research.

Conducting a national talent search, informing business organizations and others about how they can help to advance the program (i.e., raising money), selecting able students, aiding them to finance their education, and following them through their college career requires a well-trained staff and a considerable budget.

When the National Merit Scholarship Corporation was established in 1955, the administrative costs of the program had been underwritten for the following 15 years, and at least $1,000,000 had been made available for scholarships each year for the first 10 years. The total amount of money pledged by the Ford Foundation as a part of its broad program for assisting in the development and improvement of formal education was $20,000,000. The Carnegie Corporation of New York also agreed to advance $500,000 for administering the program during its first 5 years of operation; it has given an additional $250,000 to finance research during the second 5 years.

Business organizations were immediately invited to finance additional scholarships. The number of sponsors has increased year by year; by 1961 some 135 different sponsors will be offering a total of over 525 sponsored Merit Scholarships at an estimated cost to them of $2,500,000. This is in addition to the scholarships awarded by the corporation out of its resources provided through the founding grants.

The scholarship competition is conducted in this way: At the beginning of the school year all secondary schools in the United States and its territories are invited to participate in the National

Merit Scholarship Program. Participation is by school, not by individual student.

In 1960 some 15,000 schools took part in the Merit Program. There are in the United States approximately 25,000 secondary schools, but one must remember that less than one-tenth of these schools enroll over half of all students in secondary education. It is estimated that the schools which took part in the Merit Program in 1960 enroll 85% or more of all of the secondary school students in the country.

The school itself selects those of its students who will participate in the first stage of the program, a preliminary selecting test. In some schools a small number are invited to participate; in others the preliminary test is given to the entire class of third year students. Approximately 600,000 students, or about one-third of all the third year students in high school, took part in the program this past year.

The selecting test measures both the aptitude and the attainment of the student. The test is 44 pages in length and requires 3 hours for its administration. The mere act of taking the test is itself of definite educational value to the student, since it gives him the benefit of a concentrated experience in dealing with difficult intellectual tasks.

The test measures in a relatively direct fashion the complex skills required for successful work in virtually any college; it is a test of a student's readiness for high level college work. Since the skills it measures are taught in all secondary schools, the test does not favor any particular high school curriculum. Nor is the content of the test such that the student can raise his grade by frantic last-minute study; it covers too much ground for such an effort to be successful.

The scores are reported to the students by the schools. They can then be used, in conjunction with interpretative material which has been supplied to the schools, as an aid in counseling students about their future academic plans and adult careers. So no one loses by taking part in the Merit Program; there is some value for everyone.

There is considerable debate in our secondary schools about the relative importance of aptitude and achievement. Aptitude, it is supposed, is a characteristic one is born with; the schools are in no way responsible for the aptitudes of their pupils. If a person is low in intelligence or aptitude, nothing can be done for him. But achievement is a different story. Here the schools have some responsibility. The student's achievement depends upon his applying his aptitude to a specific field of endeavor. It is obvious that no one is born educated; no matter how high his intelligence is, he can learn only to the extent that he applies himself. With equal effort the very bright student will learn more than the dull student; but if the person of lesser aptitude works more diligently than the individual with greater intelligence, he may indeed climb higher than his brighter associate who has less ambition and drive.

We psychologists are largely responsible for the overemphasis which the public gives to the IQ. Frankly, the IQ is overrated. Unfortunately, parents and even many teachers regard the IQ as an infallible and crucially significant index. As a result, they ignore the importance of the many other characteristics which contribute to attainment. In the final analysis it is not how bright one is, but what one has accomplished that counts. The IQ is an empirically determined index which has certain practical values when used with appropriate caution. However, it lacks a rigorous theoretical foundation. Actually it is a composite of a number of measures of different abilities. Ability is a many-sided affair, as Dael Wolfle pointed out in the Walter V. Bingham Memorial Lecture given a year ago, and any one person may be much better at some things than at others. The IQ represents an averaging of these abilities, and so it smooths over important peaks and valleys.

The gravest danger of the IQ, however, is that it gives a grossly oversimplified picture of the organization of the mind and encourages parents, teachers, and even the students themselves to underestimate the role of effort. The relationship between the IQ and productivity, even in scholarly fields, is not as high as is generally believed.

The pupil, the teacher, and the parent should put less faith in IQ. Motivation, ambition, the ability to direct one's efforts toward a specific goal, sheer energy level, if there is such a trait—these are the characteristics which, though they are difficult to measure, determine achievement. The burning desire to excel, to be first, to be best can wisely be traded for a dozen IQ points any day.

In every aspect of life it is what one accomplishes that counts, not what his unused intelligence is, or what he might have done under other circumstances. In the Merit Program the effort of the student is considered, and all students are encouraged to apply themselves to attain greater heights in the intellectual realm.

The screening test in the Merit Program is handled by a recognized testing agency, Science Research Associates. The National Merit Scholarship Corporation does not prepare tests, sell tests, or derive any money from test sales. The corporation does specify the nature of the test it wishes and the conditions that the contractor must meet in supplying the test. To meet the heavy costs of testing, each participant pays a fee of $1.00 directly to the testing agency. If a student is unable to pay this fee, the National Merit Scholarship Corporation pays it for him.

On the basis of this screening test, a group of 35,000 students is given some type of recognition each year. Though 35,000 is a large group, it represents less than 3% of the annual crop of high school graduates. In order to have students representative of every section of the United States, the top scoring students, the Semifinalists, are chosen separately for each state. In the United States, it is the state which establishes educational policies and procedures, and consequently states differ in their educational facilities and methods. It is assumed that if we select the very best from each state, the result will be a group of superior quality, with each state contributing its proper share. Geographic representation contributes to the vitality of any national program.

Of the 35,000 students who are given recognition each year, about 10,000 are named Semifinalists. They constitute the top group, with the more populous states having more representatives and the less populous states having fewer, just as in the lower house in our Congress. California, for example, has over 750 Semifinalists while Nevada has under 15.

In addition to the Semifinalists, who constitute less than 1% of the high school graduates, a second group is selected. The 25,000 students in this group are sent Letters of Commendation encouraging them to continue with their education. The number of commended students in each state varies according to the proportion scoring high on the test nationally, without regard to the state-by-state selection of the Semifinalists. In New York, for example, in 1960 there were almost 5,000 Letters of Commendation awarded, while in three of our states, fewer than 25 students won this honor.

The Letters of Commendation were introduced in the third year of the Merit Program. At that time some skepticism was expressed as to the value of a form of recognition which is not accompanied by any financial aid. However, the results of our preliminary studies indicate that such recognition has a stimulating influence on able students. It gives them more self-confidence, it encourages them to apply themselves, and it causes them to set somewhat higher intellectual goals in life. Public recognition by itself can have a beneficial effect. When properly handled, simple means can be effective in encouraging talent.

After the 10,000 Semifinalists have been selected, they are asked to take a second test, the Scholastic Aptitude Test of the College Board. Each Semifinalist is also requested to supply certain information about himself and to have his school submit his academic record and its recommendation. Virtually all of the Semifinalists, over 97%, meet these requirements and confirm their earlier test scores. They thereby become Finalists in the program, and are eligible to receive a Merit Scholarship.

Unfortunately there is not enough money available to award a Merit Scholarship to every Finalist. The field must be narrowed even further. The recipients of the National Merit Scholarships (unsponsored scholarships made possible by the founding grants) are chosen by a committee of people skilled in exercising the kind of judgment required. This committee meets to review the list of Finalists and, on the basis of the school's recommendations, the students' test scores, academic records, and outside activities and work, to select those students from each state whom they believe to be the most highly qualified. The number of scholarships awarded in each state is roughly proportional to the high school graduates in that state in the most recent year for which statistics are available.

In addition to the unsponsored National Merit Scholarships, the corporation distributes scholarships sponsored by corporations, foundations, and individuals. Many of these sponsors leave the selection of the winners of their scholarships to the same committee which selects the winners of National Merit Scholarships. However, a sponsor may, if he wishes to do so, choose from among the Finalist group (all of whom have proved themselves to be academically qualified) those students who meet their special interests. For example, some sponsors prefer students who have an interest in science; while some prefer students residing in certain geographic areas. Many sponsors are interested in helping to finance the education of any employees' children who achieve the high status of Finalist in the Merit Program.

The secondary schools are sent complete reports on every phase of the Merit Program. In addition, the Semifinalists are listed in a book which is distributed to all colleges and other scholarship-granting agencies. Partly as a result of this distribution of names, these students receive many additional scholarship offers. About half of the Semifinalists receive either a Merit Scholarship or some other offer of financial aid.

When the students take the initial selecting test, they are asked to name the two colleges they would prefer to attend. Each college is sent a list of the students who have named that particular institution with the students' scores on the screening test. As a result, each student on the list is likely to be given greater consideration by the college for admission or financial aid than he otherwise might.

The Merit Finalists are selected without regard to their financial need. The selection is based on ability only. Thus the student selected for a Merit Scholarship may be one whose family is able to support him in college, or he may be one who needs outside help in financing his college career. On the basis of this information the amount of money to accompany the scholarship is determined. The amount depends upon the family's ability to support the student at the college of his choice.

In determining the extent of a student's need two factors are considered. The first is the amount of money the family can be expected to contribute, and the second is the cost of attending the college selected by the student. The individual stipends range from a minimum of $100 a year to a maximum of $1,500 a year. Each scholarship covers 4 years of college, assuming that the winner progresses at a normal rate and does satisfactory work.

The need factor is re-evaluated each year. If it is found that the ability of the family to support the student has changed, a new stipend is set. For example, the need of one student, the son of a business executive, was assessed at $100 a year at the time he won his scholarship. During the student's freshman year in college his father suffered a fatal heart attack. The Scholar's situation was then re-evaluated and his stipend was changed from the minimum to the maximum of $1,500 a year. In a sense, a Merit Scholarship is an insurance policy.

About a third of the Merit Scholars currently receive an annual stipend of $250 or less. At the other extreme, about 20% receive the maximum stipend of $1,500. At the present time, the average stipend is around $827 a year. Even when the amount received is only $250 or $300 a year, it can make the difference between the student's attending the college of his choice and his going to an institution which he believes to be less satisfactory. The Merit Scholarship money therefore is of major significance to most of the students.

In addition to the stipend paid to the Merit Scholar, each scholarship is accompanied by a grant to the college to be used in whatever way the college wishes. The purpose of this grant is to call public attention to the importance of assisting privately supported colleges. In 1959–60 over $750,000 was paid to the colleges. During the same year, payments to the students amounted to over $2,200,000.

Obviously, the Merit Scholar has been selected with great care from among hundreds of thousands of participants, and he is an interesting—sometimes an exciting—young person. He has scored in the top fraction, about 1%, of the high school seniors in his state. His high school academic record and recommendations are superior. His activities outside the classroom testify that he is a person of some breadth. He has been chosen as representative of the most intellectually promising of the younger generation.

In selecting scholarship winners, no consideration is given to the student's family background or social and economic status, nor is his being from the city or the country taken into account. The task is to select the most promising young people without regard to their financial need. After this has been done it is possible—as a part of the research activity, not the scholarship program as such—to check into parental occupations. As might be expected, many of the winners have parents who are well educated; the father is a physician, a lawyer, a teacher, or an executive. The interesting fact, however, is that many of the parents have more ordinary occupations.

Among the parents of the group awarded Merit Scholarships in 1959, we find barbers, bookkeepers, butchers, cab drivers, carpenters, cashiers, chauffeurs, clerks, construction workers, electricians, farmers, firemen, glass workers, junk collectors, mail carriers, mechanics, and painters. Of course some of the fathers are accountants, attorneys, business executives, clergymen, college administrators, editors, economists, physicians, and teachers. Clearly, ability is where you find it; one cannot tell from a parent's occupation or social and economic background whether or not the child will have unusual mental ability. That is why equality of educational opportunity is prized in a democracy.

The personalities of Merit Scholars are of particular interest. The public usually thinks of the very bright young student as a rather peculiar, introverted type—smaller in physique than the average, somewhat antisocial, and rather narrow in his interests.

But this image is a false one. The brainy can be brawny too. Research has shown that gifted young people are generally taller, heavier, and physically and mentally healthier than those of average intelligence. From studies of Merit Scholars we know that they have a tendency to be dominant in social situations, or more accurately, not to be submissive. They have a greater interest in people, less tendency to withdraw from social situations, and more sophistication and self-confidence than the average person. They are less tense, less anxious, less given to feelings of insecurity or depression. They show unusual originality, imagination, and resourcefulness. Most important, perhaps, researchers have characterized the Merit Scholars as "risk-takers in the field of ideas."

Where do these Scholars choose to go to college? There are well over a thousand 4-year, degree granting colleges in the United States. Since the Merit Scholars are selected from every state in the Union, it might be expected that they would spread themselves among the colleges more or less evenly. But quite the contrary is the case. A relatively small number of colleges are chosen by this high quality group of students. In the school year 1960–61, Merit Scholars are attending some four hundred different colleges and universities. One institution alone, Harvard College, has attracted almost 10% of the Merit Scholars. The 12 colleges most popular with this group attract about a third of the Merit Scholars. These are, in order: Harvard, Massachusetts Institute of Technology, Stanford, Radcliffe, Princeton, California Institute of Technology, Yale, Rice, University of Michigan, Oberlin, Swarthmore, and Cornell.

In March 1960, the 34,000 highest scoring students (who were then juniors in high school) were asked to name the one college they most wanted to attend. If any bias enters this poll, it is unknown. In this popularity contest, in which only the very brightest students have a vote, we again find a marked preference for a small number of institutions. Over one-third of these very able young men wished to attend the following colleges in the order named: Massachusetts Institute of Technology, Harvard, California Institute of Technology, Stanford, Princeton, Cornell, Yale, University of California at Berkeley, Notre Dame, and University of Michigan. Approximately one-fifth of the girls named as their first choice the following 10 institutions (listed in order of their popularity): Radcliffe, Stanford, Cornell, Wellesley, University of Michigan, University of California at Berkeley, Oberlin, Smith, Swarthmore, and Northwestern.

If we consider the number of these able students who named a particular college as a percentage of the number of students that institution admits, we get a different rank order. For the male students, California Institute of Technology was named by somewhat over four times the number of students it admits into its entering class. Next in order is Massachusetts Institute of Technology named by almost twice the number of students it admits in its freshman class. Following these two institutions come in order: Harvard, Rice, Amherst, Swarthmore, Reed, Stanford, Princeton, University of Chicago, Oberlin, Yale, Columbia, Dartmouth, Carleton, and Wesleyan University—all attracting from this very select group a vote equal to 30% or more of its entering class. If we consider the girls and rank the colleges according to their popularity with this superior group, but relative to the size of the incoming freshman class, we get this order: Swarthmore, Radcliffe, Middlebury, Rice, Stanford, Reed, Oberlin, Cornell, Carleton, Wellesley, Bryn Mawr, Smith, University of Chicago, Barnard, and Mount Holyoke.

These figures may not have any great significance. Because a student named a college as his preference, it does not necessarily follow that he is equipped intellectually, socially, or financially to attend that college, or that he would be accepted by it. We need a good deal more information before we can adequately interpret this popular vote. However, the public's interest in such polls suggests that they are worthy of some consideration. No popularity contest should be allowed to obscure the difficult problem of matching a particular student with the institution which will bring about his maximum development. In the high school-college guidance work to date too frequently the blind have been leading the blind.

One problem encountered by the Merit Program is the tendency of the public and the press to use the results of the program as an index of the value of a particular school or college. The public is apt to conclude quite erroneously that the colleges which are most popular with Merit Scholars are the best colleges for all students. Likewise, secondary schools having a large number of Finalists in the Merit Program are sometimes said to be "better" than other schools having a smaller number of Finalists. But the quality or effectiveness of a school cannot properly be judged by the number of its students who win awards in the Merit Program. All selections are made on an individual basis. The distribution of the population throughout a state, the size of a school, the native intelligence of its top students, the nature of the community where the school is located, and many other factors having nothing to do with the total effectiveness of a school can influence its number of award winners. Although it is recognized that award winners bring honor to their schools and their parents as well as to themselves, the press and the public are encouraged to judge each student individually and to refrain from comparisons of schools and colleges.

What has been the college record of Merit Scholars? The first class of Merit Scholars entered college in the fall of 1956. This initial group numbered 555, 402 (72%) of them boys and 153 (28%) girls. Of the first group, 88% of the girls and 81% of the boys have now graduated.

The outstanding record made by those who have graduated is striking. Over 60% stood in the top 10% of their class; a fifth of the group was in the top 1%. About 80% graduated with some academic honor. A number led their class—like the charming young woman who selected a college of mining and ranked first in her class, composed mainly of men, every 1 of the 4 years, graduating with high honors and incidentally gaining a husband in the process. Both are now in graduate school.

Their records in campus leadership were also outstanding. About 1 in 5 held leadership positions. Many Merit Scholars were editors of major campus publications and presidents of major student government organizations and living groups, and 20 won their letters in varsity sports.

Of these graduates, 18% of the boys and 37% of the girls have married. Slightly over 10% of the original group are still in college, because they are taking 5-year programs or because they took a year out for some reason. It is anticipated that approximately 94% of the original group will receive college degrees within 5 years after entering college.

Up to the present time slightly over 6% of this first group have left the program for one reason or another. Only 17 Merit Scholars had their scholarships terminated because of unsatisfactory work in colleges of their choice, and more than half of these students are back in college today. Fifteen Merit Scholars—eight girls and seven boys—withdrew from college while in good academic standing. Most of the girls withdrew in order to marry, and of these the majority expect to complete their degree requirements eventually.

Most of the first group of Merit Scholars are continuing their formal education beyond the bachelor's degree. Over 80% of the men and almost 60% of the women in this group plan to go on to graduate or professional schools. Eighty percent of them hold fellowships and assistantships, about half from sources outside the college or university.

The Merit Scholars obviously are a distinguished group. But what of those Finalists who did not win scholarships? We have found that over 94% go on to college. About one-half of the group are receiving some type of scholarship aid and we believe we have helped them to do so.

Of the boys who took the screening test and who ranked in the top third of all juniors in the country, about 87% are now full-time students in some college. The same is true of about 77% of the girls. Many of these students have received some scholarship help, and research shows that the higher an individual's test score, the greater the probability that he holds a scholarship.

In a recent study, one of the research staff members examined the nature of academic achievement and creative behavior in the Finalists. He finds support for the idea that the creative person (as opposed to the academic achiever) is one who is independent, intellectual, expressive, asocial, and consciously original. The mothers of creative persons are permissive and ready to accept the ideas and impulses of the young, while their fathers want them to be curious and self-reliant.

Preliminary research results suggest that these creative people are not favored by the groups who select scholarship winners. At present there are no adequate measures of potential creativity, although researchers at Merit and other places are beginning to make progress on this problem.

John Holland, Director of Research for the National Merit Scholarship Program, has written:

> It is imperative that we learn how to identify the creative person so that we can seek out and encourage such students, whatever their application form debits. They should not be penalized for their failure to play the good boy role for their high school teachers, or to satisfy the pointless demand for well-roundedness by dissipating their energies in a frenetic round of extracurricular activities and good works.

This year the Merit Program is testing some preliminary notions about creativity by selecting a small group of students from its Finalists who appear to be particularly creative.

Has the Merit Program succeeded in encouraging the recognition and development of talent? Measurement of impacts of an attack on such a broad front is difficult; we must allow more time for the dust to settle before we can take sightings. The first class of Merit Scholars is just getting under way in graduate school.

The letters of comment which reach us are overwhelmingly favorable. One official from a small college comments on the leavening effect of its six Merit Scholars:

> It is difficult to estimate the impact which these six students are having on the campus, but beyond all doubt it is terrific.

States a college president:

> The program has been successful in influencing the junior and senior high school students to approach their academic programs with seriousness of purpose which was not common a few years ago.

The chancellor of the Telluride Association, who visits many schools each year, attributes much of the high school student's changed attitude toward academic work to the influence of the Merit Program. He goes on to say:

> It is getting so a man may be a first-class scholar in a high school today and not lose social caste.

A high school principal writes:

> The Merit Program is making a critical contribution to educational thought . . . the most wonderful thing about your work is that its influence will be everlasting, for it affects profoundly the lives of boys and girls.

From the students themselves we occasionally receive some heart-warming letters. For example, a young lady from Indiana writes:

> Your program was no small factor in causing me to go to college. You see I am the first person in my family who ever indicated a desire to attend college. My parents did not even attend high school. As a result, it was not easy to convince myself and my family that college was for me. However, when I won a Certificate of Merit I was convinced I should go to college, and it helped me to win my parents over to my view.

The press's coverage of the Merit Program, increasing each year, gives evidence of the public's growing interest. Among the clippings which arrived this month was a letter to an Illinois newspaper from one of the recently graduated Merit Scholars. He says in part:

> The most significant effect of the National Merit Program is not conservation or insurance, but stimulation. National Merit winners and Finalists acquire recognition and self-realization that (1) prompts those to go to college who might not have done so otherwise, whether they received a scholarship or not; (2) encourages them to go to colleges where there is a keener competition and a greater exchange of ideas; (3) produces an incentive to work commensurate with ability. This stimulation is not a short-lived thing; it builds upon itself. The high percentage of Merit Scholars who have gone into graduate study is some evidence of this. In my own case I believe that I can say that my desire for worthwhile achievement is at present stronger than it ever was.

Evidence by testimonial, however interesting, is not convincing to the scientist. After an additional several years have gone by, an attempt will be made to obtain more accurate estimates of the impact of the Merit Program.

Because the data on talented students which have been collected are of an unparalleled quality and magnitude, the research activities of the Merit Program are particularly important and promising. Much of our research is directed toward developing new methods of scholarship selection. Heretofore, the very success of the objective scholastic aptitude and college readiness tests has discouraged experimentation with measures of other significant characteristics. It might be valuable, for example, to study such background factors as the family, the community, and the friends of able students, to ask what cultural elements in the student's background contribute to develop his talent to a productive level. The student's scholarly activity independent of classroom work may also be of greater significance than has been suspected previously.

It is difficult to assess the significance of personal characteristics not measured by the widely used scholarship selection tests, but more thorough measurement in this area may prove to be important in the identification of able persons who will be productive after college.

The Merit Program is conducting research in several other areas. The results of its research are being reported in the professional journals and through technical progress reports. This research activity, a fundamental part of the Merit Program, contributes to the health of the entire program and prevents any of the procedures from becoming frozen.

In many ways the Merit Program is a pilot venture, making explorations in an important but very complex field. By working with schools throughout the entire land, with their ablest pupils, and with the colleges which attract such students, the Merit Program gains experience in recognizing and encouraging talent. We are establishing a few guideposts and a few warning signs.

Consider an example. Talent loss is a concept which we are working to define more meaningfully. For the moment we will take it to refer to those students who are capable of doing superior college work but do not go to college. Many of these students, most of whom are girls, come from lower socioeconomic levels and from areas where college attendance is unusual. Apart from financial need, lack of motivation is the primary cause of their not going on to college. If we are to prevent this talent loss—and prevent it we must—we must identify these students in the seventh or eighth grade, perhaps even earlier.

Such talented young pupils should be introduced early in their lives to the world of ideas, to books, to scientific laboratories, and to the fun of learning. When optional routes are offered in high school, they should be guided down the path of heavy intellectual activity. Only in this way will they be both motivated and prepared to compete in the latter years of high school; only in this way can they win their share of financial help for college. Early stimulation, followed by superior educational opportunities, is the key.

Of the many things we have learned in operating the Merit Program for 5 years, the most significant is how little we know about identifying creative talent, and how much less about its proper development. The extensive folklore about able students and scholarships must be challenged, if more effective procedures are to be developed. Every sizable scholarship program should have a companion research program to find out what effect it is having, and how it can do the job better.

To discover talent we must initiate bold new methods based on sound theory and applied with imagination and practical ingenuity. Private ventures, like the Merit Program, should not be afraid to experiment, to attempt new approaches, to venture beyond established practices.

The Merit Program will continue to experiment and to learn. It will continue to encourage the public to honor intellectual excellence, to excite each community about its own able youth, to make higher education a possible goal for many students of demonstrated promise, and to create a climate favorable to intellectual excellence. It is an action program dedicated to recognizing and encouraging talent, goals which many years ago Bingham knew were among the most important ones toward which citizens of a democracy must strive. In the words of John Gardner: ". . . an undiscovered talent, a wasted skill, a misapplied ability is a threat to the capacity of a free people to survive."

*Donald W. MacKinnon*

# *The Nature and Nurture of Creative Talent*[1]

Let me say first how deeply appreciative I am of the honor of having been chosen the Walter Van Dyke Bingham Lecturer for 1962. It has for me especial meaning to be provided this opportunity to honor the memory of a man I respected so much and whose work was such a pioneering contribution to that field of psychology to which I have given most of my energies as a psychologist. I am grateful, too, for this opportunity to express to Mrs. Bingham the gratitude of all psychologists for her generosity in establishing this series of annual lectures on the discovery and development of exceptional abilities and capacities. Our literature has been greatly enriched by the lectures which she has made possible.

I should like also to congratulate Yale University for having been chosen this year as the institution to be honored for its contributions to the study of talent, and to thank all those who have made such pleasant arrangements for this occasion.

1. This paper is based on the Walter Van Dyke Bingham Lecture given at Yale University, New Haven, Connecticut, April 11, 1962. It was first published in the *American Psychologist,* 1962, vol. 17, no. 7 (July), pp. 484–495.

There is a story, first told I believe by Mark Twain which, had Dr. Bingham known it, would have been, I am sure, one of his favorites. It is about a man who sought the greatest general who had ever lived. Upon inquiring as to where this individual might be found, he was told that the person he sought had died and gone to Heaven. At the Pearly Gates he informed St. Peter of the purpose of his quest, whereupon St. Peter pointed to a soul nearby. "But that," protested the inquirer, "isn't the greatest of all generals. I knew that person when he lived on earth, and he was only a cobbler." "I know that," replied St. Peter, "but if he had been a general he would have been the greatest of them all."

Dr. Bingham spent his life worrying about cobblers who might have been generals and indeed about all those who fail to become what they are capable of becoming because neither they nor others recognize their potentialities and nourish their realization. Dr. Bingham was one of the first to insist that it is not enough to recognize creative talent after it has come to expression. He reminded us that it is our task as psychologists and as educators either through our insights or through the use of validated predictors to discover talent when it is still potential and to provide that kind of social climate and intellectual environment which will facilitate its development and expression.

Whatever light I shall be able to shed on the nature and nurture of creative talent comes in the main from findings of researches carried on during the last six years in the Institute of Personality Assessment and Research on the Berkeley campus of the University of California, and supported in large part by the Carnegie Corporation of New York.

In undertaking such a study one of our first tasks was to decide what we would consider creativity to be. This was necessary, first, because creativity has been so variously described and defined, and second, because only when we had come to agreement as to how we would conceive creativity would we be in a position to know what kinds of persons we would want to study.

We came easily to agreement that true creativeness fulfills at least three conditions. It involves a response or an idea that is novel or at the very least statistically infrequent. But novelty or originality of thought or action, while a necessary aspect of creativity, is not sufficient. If a response is to lay claim to being a part of the creative process, it must to some extent be adaptive to, or of, reality. It must serve to solve a problem, fit a situation, or accomplish some recognizable goal. And, thirdly, true creativeness involves a sustaining of the original insight, an evaluation and elaboration of it, a developing of it to the full.

Creativity, from this point of view, is a process extended in time and characterized by originality, adaptiveness, and realization. It may be brief, as in a musical improvisation, or it may involve a considerable span of years as was required for Darwin's creation of the theory of evolution.

The acceptance of such a conception of creativity had two important consequences for our researches. It meant that we would not seek to study creativity while it was still potential but only after it had been realized and had found expression in clearly identifiable creative products—buildings designed by architects, mathematical proofs developed by mathematicians, and the published writings of poets and novelists. Our conception of creativity forced us further to reject as indicators or criteria of creativeness the performance of individuals on so-called tests of creativity. While tests of this sort, that require that the subject think, for example, of unusual uses for common objects and the consequences of unusual events, may indeed measure the infrequency or originality of a subject's ideas in response to specific test items, they fail to reveal the extent to which the subject faced with real life problems is likely to come up with solutions that are novel and adaptive and which he will be motivated to apply in all of their ramifications.

Having thus determined that we would limit our researches to the study of persons who had already demonstrated a high level of creative work, we were still confronted with the problem of deciding from which fields of creative endeavor we would seek to recruit our subjects.

The fields which we finally sampled were those of creative writing, architecture, mathematics, industrial research, physical science, and engineering.

If one considers these activities in relation to the distinction often made between artistic and scientific creativity, it may be noted that we have sampled both of these domains as well as overlapping domains of creative striving which require that the practitioner be at one and the same time both artist and scientist.

Artistic creativity, represented in our studies by the work of poets, novelists, and essayists, results in products that are clearly expressions of the creator's inner states, his needs, perceptions, motivations, and the like. In this type of creativity, the creator externalizes something of himself into the public field.

In scientific creativity, the creative product is unrelated to the creator as a person, who in his creative work acts largely as a mediator between externally defined needs and goals. In this kind of creativeness, the creator, represented in our studies by industrial researchers, physical scientists, and engineers, simply operates on some aspect of his environment in such a manner as to produce a novel and appropriate product, but he adds little of himself or of his style as a person to the resultant.

Domains of creative striving in which the practitioner must be both artist and scientist were represented in our researches by mathematicians and architects. Mathematicians contribute to science, yet in a very real sense their important creative efforts are as much as anything else personal cosmologies in which they express themselves as does the artist in his creations. So, too, in architecture, creative products are both an expression of the architect and thus a very personal product, and at the same time an impersonal meeting of the demands of an external problem.

If in reporting the findings of our researches I draw most heavily upon data obtained from our study of architects (MacKinnon, 1962), it is for two reasons. First, it is the study for which, in collaboration with Wallace B. Hall, I have assumed primary responsibility. Second, it is in architects, of all our samples, that we can expect to find what is most generally characteristic of creative persons. Architecture, as a field of creative endeavor, requires that the successful practitioner be both artist and scientist—artist in that his designs must fulfill the demands of "Delight," and scientist in that they must meet the demands of "Firmnesse" and "Commodity," to use the words of Sir Henry Wotton (1624). But surely, one can hardly think that the requirements of effective architecture are limited to these three demands. The successful and effective architect must, with the skill of a juggler, combine, reconcile, and exercise the diverse skills of businessman, lawyer, artist, engineer, and advertising man, as well as those of author and journalist, psychiatrist, educator, and psychologist. In what other profession can one expect better to observe the multifarious expressions of creativity?

It should be clear that any attempt to discover the distinguishing traits of creative persons can succeed only in so far as some group of qualified experts can agree upon who are the more and who are the less creative workers in a given field of endeavor. In our study of architects we began by asking a panel of experts—five professors of architecture, each working independently—to nominate the 40 most creative architects in the United States. All told they supplied us with 86 names instead of the 40 they would have mentioned had there been perfect agreement among them. While 13 of the 86 architects were nominated by all five panel members, and 9 nominated by four, 11 by three, and 13 by two,

40 were individual nominations each proposed by a single panel member.

The agreement among experts is not perfect, yet far greater than one might have expected. Later we asked 11 editors of the American architectural journals, *Architectural Forum, Architectural Record,* the *Journal of the American Institute of Architects,* and *Progressive Architecture,* to rate the creativity of the 64 of the nominated architects whom we invited to participate in the study. Still later we asked the 40 nominated creative architects who actually accepted our invitation to be studied to rate the creativity of the invited 64 architects, themselves included. Since the editors' ratings of the creativity of the architects correlated +.88 with the architects' own ratings, it is clear that under certain conditions and for certain groups it is possible to obtain remarkable agreement about the relative creativeness of individual members of a profession and thus meet the first requirement for an effective study of creative persons.

A second requirement for the successful establishment of the traits of creative individuals is their willingness to make themselves available for study. Our hope was to win the cooperation of each person whom we invited to participate in the research, but as I have already indicated in the case of the architects, to obtain 40 acceptances, 64 invitations had to be sent out.

The invitation to this group, as to all the creative groups which we have studied, was to come to Berkeley for a weekend of intensive study in the Institute of Personality Assessment and Research. There, in groups of tens, they have been studied by the variety of means which constitute the assessment method—by problem-solving experiments; by tests designed to discover what a person does not know or is unable or unwilling to reveal about himself; by tests and questionnaires that permit a person to manifest various aspects of his personality and to express his attitudes, interests, and values; by searching interviews that cover the life history and reveal the present structure of the person; and by specially contrived social situations of a stressful character which call for the subject's best behavior in a socially defined role.

The response of creative persons to the invitation to reveal themselves under such trying circumstances has varied considerably. At the one extreme there have been those who replied in anger at what they perceived to be the audacity of psychologists in presuming to study so ineffable and mysterious a thing as the creative process and so sensitive a being as a creative person. At the other extreme were those who replied courteously and warmheartedly, welcoming the invitation to be studied, and manifesting even an eagerness to contribute to a better understanding of the creative person and the creative process.

Here we were face to face with a problem that plagues us in all our researches: Are those who are willing to be assessed different in important ways from those who refuse? With respect to psychological traits and characteristics we can never know. But with respect to differences in creativeness, if any, between the 40 who accepted and the 24 who declined our invitation, we know that the two groups are indistinguishable. When the nominating panel's ratings of creativity were converted to standard scores and the means for the 24 versus the 40 were compared, they were found to be identical. When the editors' ratings were similarly converted to standard scores, the mean for the nonassessed group was slightly higher (51.9) than for the assessed sample (48.7), but the difference is not statistically significant.

Certainly we cannot claim to have assessed the 40 most creative architects in the country, or the most creative of any of the groups we have studied; but it is clear that we have studied a highly creative group of architects indistinguishable in their creativity from the group of 24 who declined to be studied, and so with the other groups too.

A third requirement for the successful determination of the traits of highly creative persons in any field of endeavor is that the profession be widely sampled beyond those nominated as most creative, for the distinguishing characteristics of the restricted sample might well have nothing to do with their creativeness. Instead they might be traits characterizing all members of the profession whether creative or not, distinguishing the professional group as a whole but in no sense limited or peculiar to its highly creative members. In the case of the architects, to use them once again as an example, two additional samples were recruited for study, both of which matched the highly creative sample (whom I shall now call Architects I) with respect to age and geographic location of practice. The first supplementary sample (Architects II) had had at least two years of work experience and association with one of the originally nominated creative architects. The second additional sample (Architects III) was composed of architects who had never worked with any of the nominated creatives.

By selecting three samples in this manner, we hoped to tap a range of talent sufficiently wide to be fairly representative of the profession as a whole; and we appear to have succeeded. The mean rating of creativity for each of the three groups—the ratings having been made on a nine-point scale by six groups of architects and experts on architecture—was for Architects I, 5.46; for Architects II, 4.25; and for Architects III, 3.54, the differences in mean ratings between each group being statistically highly significant.

So much for method and research design. I turn now to a discussion of the nature of creative talent as it has been revealed to us in our researches.

Persons who are highly creative are inclined to have a good opinion of themselves, as evidenced by the large number of favorable adjectives which they use in self-description and by the relatively high scores they earn on a scale which measures basic acceptance of the self. Indeed, there is here a paradox, for in addition to their favorable self-perceptions the very basic self-acceptance of the more creative persons often permits them to speak more frankly and thus more critically and in unusual ways about themselves. It is clear, too, that the self-images of the more creative differ from the self-images of the less creative. For example, Architects I, in contrast to Architects II and III, more often describe themselves as inventive, determined, independent, individualistic, enthusiastic, and industrious. In striking contrast Architects II and III more often than Architects I describe themselves as responsible, sincere, reliable, dependable, clear thinking, tolerant, and understanding. In short, where creative architects more often stress their inventiveness, independence, and individuality, their enthusiasm, determination, and industry, less creative members of the profession are impressed by their virtue and good character and by their rationality and sympathetic concern for others.

The discrepancies between their descriptions of themselves as they are and as they would ideally be are remarkably alike for all architects regardless of their level of creativeness. All three groups reveal themselves as desiring more personal attractiveness, self-confidence, maturity, and intellectual competence, a higher level of energy, and better social relations. As for differences, however, Architects I would ideally be more sensitive, while both Architects II and III wish for opposites if not incompatibles; they would ideally be more original but at the same time more self-controlled and disciplined.

As for the relation between intelligence and creativity, save for the mathematicians where there is a low positive correlation between intelligence and the level of creativeness, we have found within our creative samples essentially zero relationship between the two variables, and this is not due to a narrow restriction in range of intelligence. Among creative architects who have a mean score of 113 on the Terman Concept Mastery Test (1956), individual scores range widely from 39 to 179, yet scores on this measure of intelligence correlate −.08 with rated creativity. Over the whole range of intelligence and creativity there is, of course, a positive relationship between the two variables. No feeble-minded subjects have shown up in any of our creative groups. It is clear, however, that above a certain required minimum level of intelligence which varies from field to field and in some instances may be surprisingly low, being more intelligent does not guarantee a corresponding increase in creativeness. It just is not true that the more intelligent person is necessarily the more creative one.

In view of the often asserted close association of genius with insanity it is also of some interest to inquire into the psychological health of our creative subjects. To this end we can look at their profiles on the Minnesota Multiphasic Personality Inventory (MMPI) (Hathaway & McKinley, 1945), a test originally developed to measure tendencies toward the major psychiatric disturbances that man is heir to: depression, hysteria, paranoia, schizophrenia, and the like. On the eight scales which measure the strength of these dispositions in the person, our creative subjects earn scores which, on the average, are some 5 to 10 points above the general population's average score of 50. It must be noted, however, that elevated scores of this degree on these scales do not have the same meaning for the personality functioning of persons who, like our subjects, are getting along well in their personal lives and professional careers, that they have for hospitalized patients. The manner in which creative subjects describe themselves on this test as well as in the life history psychiatric interview is less suggestive of psychopathology than it is of good intellect, complexity and richness of personality, general lack of defensiveness, and candor in self-description—in other words, an openness to experience and especially to experience of one's inner life. It must also be noted, however, that in the self-reports and in the MMPI profiles of many of our creative subjects, one can find rather clear evidence of psychopathology, but also evidence of adequate control mechanisms, as the success with which they live their productive and creative lives testifies.

However, the most striking aspect of the MMPI profiles of all our male creative groups is an extremely high peak on the *Mf* (femininity) scale. This tendency for creative males to score relatively high on femininity is also demonstrated on the Fe (femininity) scale of the California Psychological Inventory (CPI) (Gough, 1957) and on the masculinity-femininity scale of the Strong Vocational Interest Blank (Strong, 1959). Scores on the latter scale (where high score indicates more masculinity) correlate −.49 with rated creativity.

The evidence is clear: The more creative a person is the more he reveals an openness to his own feelings and emotions, a sensitive intellect and understanding self-awareness, and wide-ranging interests including many which in the American culture are thought of as feminine. In the realm of sexual identification and interests, our creative subjects appear to give more expression to the feminine side of their nature than do less creative persons. In the language of the Swiss psychologist, Carl G. Jung (1956), creative persons are not so completely identified with their masculine *persona* roles as to blind themselves to or to deny expression to the more feminine traits of the *anima*. For some, to be sure, the balance between masculine and feminine traits, interests, and identification, is a precarious one, and for several of our subjects it would appear that their presently achieved reconciliation of these opposites of their nature has been barely effected and only after considerable psychic stress and turmoil.

The perceptiveness of the creative and his openness to richness and complexity of experience is strikingly revealed on the Barron-Welsh Art Scale of the Welsh Figure Preference Test

(Welsh, 1959), which presents to the subject a set of 62 abstract line drawings which range from simple and symmetrical figures to complex and asymmetrical ones. In the original study (Barron & Welsh, 1952) which standardized this scale, some 80 painters from New York, San Francisco, New Orleans, Chicago, and Minneapolis showed a marked preference for the complex and asymmetrical, or, as they often referred to them, the vital and dynamic figures. A contrasting sample of nonartists revealed a marked preference for the simple and symmetrical drawings.

All creative groups we have studied have shown a clear preference for the complex and asymmetrical, and in general the more creative a person is the stronger is this preference. Similarly, in our several samples, scores on an Institute scale which measures the preference for perceptual complexity are significantly correlated with creativity. In the sample of architects the correlation is +.48.

Presented with a large selection of one-inch squares of varicolored poster board and asked to construct within a 30-minute period a pleasing, completely filled-in 8″ × 10″ mosaic (Hall, 1958), some subjects select the fewest colors possible (one used only one color, all white) while others seek to make order out of the largest possible number, using all of the 22 available colors. And, again citing results from the architects, there is a significant though low positive correlation of +.38 between the number of colors a subject chooses and his creativity as rated by the experts.

If one considers for a moment the meaning of these preferences on the art scale, on the mosaic test, and on the scale that measures preference for perceptual complexity, it is clear that creative persons are especially disposed to admit complexity and even disorder into their perceptions without being made anxious by the resulting chaos. It is not so much that they like disorder per se, but that they prefer the richness of the disordered to the stark barrenness of the simple. They appear to be challenged by disordered multiplicity which arouses in them a strong need which in them is serviced by a superior capacity to achieve the most difficult and far-reaching ordering of the richness they are willing to experience.

The creative person's openness to experience is further revealed on the Myers-Briggs Type Indicator (Myers, 1958), a test based largely upon Carl G. Jung's (1923) theory of psychological functions and types.

Employing the language of the test, though in doing so I oversimplify both it and the theory upon which it is based, one might say that whenever a person uses his mind for any purpose, he performs either an act of perception (he becomes aware of something) or an act of judgment (he comes to a conclusion about something). And most persons tend to show a rather consistent preference for and greater pleasure in one or the other of these, preferring either to perceive or to judge, though everyone both perceives and judges.

An habitual preference for the judging attitude may lead to some prejudging and at the very least to the living of a life that is orderly, controlled, and carefully planned. A preference for the perceptive attitude results in a life that is more open to experience both from within and from without, and characterized by flexibility and spontaneity. A judging type places more emphasis upon the control and regulation of experience, while a perceptive type is inclined to be more open and receptive to all experience.

The majority of our creative writers, mathematicians, and architects are perceptive types. Only among research scientists do we find the majority to be judging types, and even in this group it is interesting to note that there is a positive correlation (+.25) between a scientist's preference for perception and his rated creativity as a scientific researcher. For architects, preference for perception correlates +.41 with rated creativity.

The second preference measured by the Type Indicator is for one of two types of perception: sense perception or sensation, which is a direct becoming aware of things by way of the senses versus intuitive perception or intuition, which is an indirect perception of the deeper meanings and possibilities inherent in things and situations. Again, everyone senses and intuits, but preliminary norms for the test suggest that in the United States three out of four persons show a preference for sense perception, concentrating upon immediate sensory experience and centering their attention upon existing facts. The one out of every four who shows a preference for intuitive perception, on the other hand, looks expectantly for a bridge or link between that which is given and present and that which is not yet thought of, focusing habitually upon possibilities.

One would expect creative persons not to be bound to the stimulus and the object but to be ever alert to the as-yet-not-realized. And that is precisely the way they show themselves to be on the Type Indicator. In contrast to an estimated 25% of the general population who are intuitive, 90% of the creative writers, 92% of the mathematicians, 93% of the research scientists, and 100% of the architects are intuitive as measured by this test.

In judging or evaluating experience, according to the underlying Jungian theory of the test, one makes use of thought or of feeling; thinking being a logical process aimed at an impersonal fact-weighing analysis, while feeling is a process of appreciation and evaluation of things that gives them a personal and subjective value. A preference for thinking or for feeling appears to be less related to one's creativity as such than to the type of materials or concepts with which one deals. Of our creative groups, writers prefer feeling, mathematicians, research scientists, and engineers prefer thinking, while architects split fifty-fifty in their preference for one or the other of the two functions.

The final preference in Jungian typology and on the test is the well-known one between introversion and extraversion. Approximately two-thirds of all our creative groups score as introverts, though there is no evidence that introverts as such are more creative than extraverts.

Turning to preferences among interests and values, one would expect the highly creative to be rather different from less creative people, and there is clear evidence that they are.

On the Strong Vocational Interest Blank, which measures the similarity of a person's expressed interests with the known interests of individuals successful in a number of occupations and professions, all of our creative subjects have shown, with only slight variation from group to group, interests similar to those of the psychologist, author-journalist, lawyer, architect, artist, and musician, and interests unlike those of the purchasing agent, office man, banker, farmer, carpenter, veterinarian, and interestingly enough, too, policeman and mortician. Leaving aside any consideration of the specific interests thus revealed we may focus our attention on the inferences that may be drawn from this pattern of scores which suggest that creative persons are relatively uninterested in small details, or in facts for their own sake, and more concerned with their meanings and implications, possessed of considerable cognitive flexibility, verbally skillful, interested in communicating with others and accurate in so doing, intellectually curious, and relatively disinterested in policing either their own impulses and images or those of others.

On the Allport-Vernon-Lindzey Study of Values (1951), a test designed to measure in the individual the relative strength of the six values of men as these values have been conceptualized and described by the German psychologist and educator, Eduard Spranger (1928), namely, the theoretical, economic, esthetic, social, political, and religious values, all of our creative groups have as their highest values the theoretical and the esthetic.

For creative research scientists the theoretical value is the highest, closely followed by the esthetic. For creative architects the highest value is the esthetic, with the theoretical value almost as high. For creative mathematicians, the two values are both high and approximately equally strong.

If, as the authors of the test believe, there is some incompatibility and conflict between the theoretical value with its cognitive and rational concern with truth and the esthetic value with its emotional concern with form and beauty, it would appear that the creative person has the capacity to tolerate the tension that strong opposing values create in him, and in his creative striving he effects some reconciliation of them. For the truly creative person it is not sufficient that problems be solved; there is the further demand that the solutions be elegant. He seeks both truth and beauty.

A summary description of the creative person—especially of the creative architect—as he reveals himself in his profile on the California Psychological Inventory (Gough, 1957) reads as follows:

> He is dominant (Do scale); possessed of those qualities and attributes which underlie and lead to the achievement of social status (Cs); poised, spontaneous, and self-confident in personal and social interaction (Sp); though not of an especially sociable or participative temperament (low Sy); intelligent, outspoken, sharp-witted, demanding, aggressive, and self-centered; persuasive and verbally fluent, self-confident and self-assured (Sa); and relatively uninhibited in expressing his worries and complaints (low Wb).
>
> He is relatively free from conventional restraints and inhibitions (low So and Sc), not preoccupied with the impression which he makes on others and thus perhaps capable of great independence and autonomy (low Gi), and relatively

ready to recognize and admit self-views that are unusual and unconventional (low Cm).

He is strongly motivated to achieve in situations in which independence in thought and action are called for (Ai). But, unlike his less creative colleagues, he is less inclined to strive for achievement in settings where conforming behavior is expected or required (Ac). In efficiency and steadiness of intellectual effort (Ie), however, he does not differ from his fellow workers.

Finally, he is definitely more psychologically minded (Py), more flexible (Fx), and possessed of more femininity of interests (Fe) than architects in general.

There is one last finding that I wish to present, one that was foreshadowed by a discovery of Dr. Bingham in one of his attempts to study creativity. The subject of his study was Amy Lowell, a close friend of his and Mrs. Bingham's, with whom he discussed at length the birth and growth of her poems, seeking insight into the creative processes of her mind. He also administered to her a word association test and "found that she gave a higher proportion of unique responses than those of any one outside a mental institution" (Bingham, Millicent Todd, 1953, p. 11). We, too, administered a word association test to our subjects and found the unusualness of mental associations one of the best predictors of creativity, and especially so when associations given by no more than 1% to 10% of the population, using the Minnesota norms (Russell & Jenkins, 1954), are weighted more heavily than those given by less than 1% of the population. Among architects, for example, this weighted score is for Architects I, 204; Architects II, 128; and Architects III, 114; while for the total sample this measure of unusualness of mental associations correlates +.50 with rated creativity.

And Dr. Bingham, like us, found that there are certain hazards in attempting to study a creative poet. His searchings were rewarded by a poem Amy Lowell later wrote which was first entitled "To the Impudent Psychologist" and published posthumously with the title "To a Gentleman who wanted to see the first drafts of my poems in the interest of psychological research into the workings of the creative mind." We, I must confess, were treated somewhat less kindly by one of our poets who, after assessment, published an article entitled "My Head Gets Tooken Apart" (Rexroth, 1959).

Having described the overall design of our studies, and having presented a selection of our findings which reveal at least some aspects of the nature of creative talent, I turn now, but with considerably less confidence, to the question as to how we can early identify and best encourage the development of creative potential. Our findings concerning the characteristics of highly creative persons are by now reasonably well established, but their implications for the nurture of creative talent are far from clear.

It is one thing to discover the distinguishing characteristics of mature, creative, productive individuals. It is quite another matter to conclude that the traits of creative persons observed several years after school and college characterized these same individuals when they were students. Nor can we be certain that finding these same traits in youngsters today will identify those with creative potential. Only empirical, longitudinal research, which we do not yet have, can settle such issues. Considering, however, the nature of the traits which discriminate creative adults from their noncreative peers, I would venture to guess that most students with creative potential have personality structures congruent with, though possibly less sharply delineated than, those of mature creatives.

Our problem is further complicated by the fact that though

our creative subjects have told us about their experiences at home, in school, and in college, and about the forces and persons and situations which, as they see it, nurtured their creativeness, these are, after all, self-reports subject to the misperceptions and self-deceptions of all self-reports. Even if we were to assume that their testimony is essentially accurate we would still have no assurance that the conditions in the home, in school, and in society, the qualities of interpersonal relations between instructor and student, and the aspects of the teaching-learning process which would appear to have contributed to creative development a generation ago would facilitate rather than inhibit creativity if these same factors were created in today's quite different world and far different educational climate.

In reporting upon events and situations in the life histories of our subjects which appear to have fostered their creative potential and independent spirit, I shall again restrict myself to architects. One finds in their histories a number of circumstances which, in the early years, could well have provided an opportunity as well as the necessity for developing the secure sense of personal autonomy and zestful commitment to their profession which so markedly characterize them.

What appears most often to have characterized the parents of these future creative architects was an extraordinary respect for the child and confidence in his ability to do what was appropriate. Thus they did not hesitate to grant him rather unusual freedom in exploring his universe and in making decisions for himself—and this early as well as late. The expectation of the parent that the child would act independently but reasonably and responsibly appears to have contributed immensely to the latter's sense of personal autonomy which was to develop to such a marked degree.

The obverse side of this was that there was often a lack of intense closeness with one or both of the parents. Most often this appeared in relation to the father rather than to the mother, but often it characterized the relationship with both parents. There were not strong emotional ties of either a positive or a negative sort between parent and child, but neither was there the type of relationship that fosters overdependency nor the type that results in severe rejection. Thus, if there was a certain distance in the relationship between child and parent, it had a liberating effect so far as the child was concerned. If he lacked something of the emotional closeness which some children experience with their parents, he was also spared that type of psychological exploitation that is so frequently seen in the life histories of clinical patients.

Closely related to this factor of some distance between parent and child were ambiguities in identification with the parents. In place of the more usual clear identification with one parent, there was a tendency for the architects to have identified either with both parents or with neither. It was not that the child's early milieu was a deprived one so far as models for identification and the promotion of ego ideals were concerned. It was rather that the larger familial sphere presented the child with a plentiful supply of diverse and effective models—in addition to the mother and father, grandfathers, uncles, and others who occupied prominent and responsible positions within their community—with whom important identifications could be made. Whatever the emotional interaction between father and son, whether distant, harmonious, or turbulent, the father presented a model of effective and resourceful behavior in an exceptionally demanding career. What is perhaps more significant, though, is the high incidence of distinctly autonomous mothers among families of the creative architects, who led active lives with interests and sometimes careers of their own apart from their husbands'.

Still other factors which would appear to have contributed to the development of the marked personal autonomy of our subjects were the types of discipline and religious training which they received, which suggest that within the family there existed clear standards of conduct and ideas as to what was right and wrong but at the same time an expectation if not requirement of active exploration and internalization of a framework of personal conduct. Discipline was almost always consistent and predictable. In most cases there were rules, family standards, and parental injunctions which were known explicitly by the children and seldom infringed. In nearly half the cases, corporal punishment was not employed and in only a few instances was the punishment harsh or cruel.

As for religious practices, the families of the creative architects showed considerable diversity, but what was most widely emphasized was the development of personal ethical codes rather than formal religious practices. For one-third of the families formal religion was important for one parent or for both, but in two-thirds of the families formal religion was either unimportant or practiced only perfunctorily. For the majority of the families, in which emphasis was placed upon the development of one's own ethical code, it is of interest to inquire into the values that were most stressed. They were most often values related to integrity (e.g., forthrightness, honesty, respect for others), quality (e.g., pride, diligence, joy in work, development of talent), intellectual and cultural endeavor, success and ambition, and being respectable and doing the right thing.

The families of the more creative architects tended to move more frequently, whether within a single community, or from community to community, or even from country to country. This, combined with the fact that the more creative architects as youngsters were given very much more freedom to roam and to explore widely, provided for them an enrichment of experience both cultural and personal which their less creative peers did not have.

But the frequent moving appears also to have resulted frequently in some estrangement of the family from its immediate neighborhood. And it is of interest that in almost every case in which the architect reported that his family differed in its behavior and values from those in the neighborhood, the family was different in showing greater cultural, artistic, and intellectual interests and pursuits.

To what extent this sort of cultural dislocation contributed to the frequently reported experiences of aloneness, shyness, isolation, and solitariness during childhood and adolescence, with little or no dating during adolescence, or to what extent these experiences stemmed from a natural introversion of interests and unusual sensitivity, we cannot say. They were doubtless mutually reinforcing factors in stimulating the young architect's awareness of his own inner life and his growing interest in his artistic skills and his ideational, imaginal, and symbolic processes.

Almost without exception, the creative architects manifested very early considerable interest and skill in drawing and painting. And also, with almost no exception, one or both of the parents were of artistic temperament and considerable skill. Often it was the mother who in the architect's early years fostered his artistic potentialities by her example as well as by her instruction. It is especially interesting to note, however, that while the visual and artistic abilities and interests of the child were encouraged and rewarded, these interests and abilities were, by and large, allowed to develop at their own speed, and this pace varied considerably among the architects. There was not an anxious concern on the part of the parents about the skills and abilities of the child. What is perhaps most significant was the widespread definite lack of strong pressures from the parents toward a particular career. And this was true both for pressures away from architecture as well as for pressures toward architecture by parents who were themselves architects.

The several aspects of the life history which I have described were first noted by Kenneth Craik in the protocols for the highly creative Architects I. Subsequently, in reading the protocols for Architects II and III as well as Architects I, a credit of one point for the presence of each of the factors was assigned and the total for each person taken as a score. The correlation of these life history scores with rated creativity of the architects is +.36, significant beyond the .005 level of confidence.

And now I turn finally to a consideration of the implications of the nature of creative talent for the nurturing of it in school and college through the processes of education.

Our findings concerning the relations of intelligence to creativity suggest that we may have overestimated in our educational system the role of intelligence in creative achievement. If our expectation is that a child of a given intelligence will not respond creatively to a task which confronts him, and especially if we make this expectation known to the child, the probability that he will respond creatively is very much reduced. And later on, such a child, now grown older, may find doors closed to him so that he is definitely excluded from certain domains of learning. There is increasing reason to believe that in selecting students for special training of their talent we may have overweighted the role of intelligence either by setting the cutting point for selection on the intellective dimension too high or by assuming that regardless of other factors the student with the higher IQ is the more promising one and should consequently be chosen. Our data suggest, rather, that if a person has the minimum of intelligence required for mastery of a field of knowledge, whether he performs creatively or banally in that field will be crucially determined by nonintellective factors. We would do well then to pay more attention in the future than we have in the past to the nurturing of those nonintellective traits which in our studies have been shown to be intimately associated with creative talent.

There is the openness of the creative person to experience both from within and from without which suggests that whether we be parent or teacher we should use caution in setting limits upon what those whom we are nurturing experience and express.

Discipline and self-control are necessary. They must be learned if one is ever to be truly creative, but it is important that they not be overlearned. Furthermore, there is a time and place for their learning, and having been learned they should be used flexibly, not rigidly or compulsively.

If we consider this specifically with reference to the attitudes of perceiving and judging, everyone must judge as well as perceive. It is not a matter of using one to the exclusion of the other, but a question of how each is used and which is preferred. The danger for one's creative potential is not the judging or evaluating of one's experience but that one prejudges, thus excluding from perception large areas of experience. The danger in all parental instruction, as in all academic instruction, is that new ideas and new possibilities of action are criticized too soon and too often. Training in criticism is obviously important and so widely recognized that I need not plead its case. Rather I would urge that, if we wish to nurture creative potential, an equal emphasis be placed on perceptiveness, discussing with our students as well as with our children, at least upon occasion, the most fantastic of ideas and possibilities. It is the duty of parents to communicate and of professors to profess what they judge to be true, but it is no less their duty by example to encourage in their children and in their students an openness to all ideas and especially to those which most challenge and threaten their own judgments.

The creative person, as we have seen, is not only open to experience, but intuitive about it. We can train students to be accurate in their perceptions, and this, too, is a characteristic of the creative. But can we train them to be intuitive, and if so how?

I would suggest that rote learning, learning of facts for their own sake, repeated drill of material, too much emphasis upon facts unrelated to other facts, and excessive concern with memorizing, can all strengthen and reinforce sense perception. On the other hand, emphasis upon the transfer of training from one subject to another, the searching for common principles in terms of which facts from quite different domains of knowledge can be related, the stressing of analogies, and similes, and metaphors, a seeking for symbolic equivalents of experience in the widest possible number of sensory and imaginal modalities, exercises in imaginative play, training in retreating from the facts in order to see them in larger perspective and in relation to more aspects of the larger context thus achieved—these and still other emphases in learning would, I believe, strengthen the disposition to intuitive perception as well as intuitive thinking.

If the widest possible relationships among facts are to be established, if the structure of knowledge (Bruner, 1960) is to be grasped, it is necessary that the student have a large body of facts which he has learned as well as a large array of reasoning skills which he has mastered. You will see, then, that what I am proposing is not that in teaching one disdain acute and accurate sense perception, but that one use it to build upon, leading the student always to an intuitive understanding of that which he experiences.

The independence of thought and action which our subjects reveal in the assessment setting appears to have long characterized them. It was already manifest in high school, though, according to their reports, tending to increase in college and thereafter.

In college our creative architects earned about a B average.

In work and courses which caught their interest they could turn in an A performance, but in courses that failed to strike their imagination, they were quite willing to do no work at all. In general, their attitude in college appears to have been one of profound skepticism. They were unwilling to accept anything on the mere say-so of their instructors. Nothing was to be accepted on faith or because it had behind it the voice of authority. Such matters might be accepted, but only after the student on his own had demonstrated their validity to himself. In a sense, they were rebellious, but they did not run counter to the standards out of sheer rebelliousness. Rather, they were spirited in their disagreement and one gets the impression that they learned most from those who were not easy with them. But clearly many of them were not easy to take. One of the most rebellious, but, as it turned out, one of the most creative, was advised by the Dean of his School to quit because he had no talent; and another, having been failed in his design dissertation which attacked the stylism of the faculty, took his degree in the art department.

These and other data should remind all of us who teach that creative students will not always be to our liking. This will be due not only to their independence in situations in which nonconformity may be seriously disruptive of the work of others, but because, as we have seen, more than most they will be experiencing large quantities of tension produced in them by the richness of their experience and the strong opposites of their nature. In struggling to reconcile these opposites and in striving to achieve creative solutions to the difficult problems which they have set themselves they will often show that psychic turbulence which is so characteristic of the creative person. If, however, we can only recognize the sources of their disturbance, which often enough will result in behavior disturbing to us, we may be in a better position to support and encourage them in their creative striving.

### *References*

Allport, G. W., Vernon, P. E., & Lindzey, G. *Study of values: manual of directions.* (Rev. ed.) Boston: Houghton Mifflin, 1951.

Barron, F., & Welsh, G. S. Artistic perception as a possible factor in personality style: its measurement by a figure preference test. *J. Psychol.*, 1952, 33, 199–203.

Bingham, Millicent Todd. Beyond psychology. In *Homo sapiens auduboniensis: a tribute to Walter Van Dyke Bingham.* New York: National Audubon Society, 1953, pp. 5–29.

Bruner, J. S. *The process of education.* Cambridge, Mass.: Harvard Univer. Press, 1960.

Gough, H. G. *California Psychological Inventory manual.* Palo Alto, Calif.: Consulting Psychologists Press, 1957.

Hall, W. B. The development of a technique for assessing aesthetic predispositions and its application to a sample of professional research scientists. Paper read at Western Psychological Association, Monterey, California, April 1958.

Hathaway, S. R., & McKinley, J. C. *Minnesota Multiphasic Personality Inventory.* New York: Psychological Corporation, 1945.

Jung, C. G. *Psychological types.* New York: Harcourt, Brace, 1923.

Jung, C. G. *Two essays on analytical psychology.* New York: Meridian, 1956.

MacKinnon, D. W. The personality correlates of creativity: a study of American architects. In G. S. Nielsen (ed.), *Proceedings of the XIV International Congress of Applied Psychology, Copenhagen 1961.* Vol. 2. Copenhagen: Munksgaard, 1962, pp. 11–39.

Myers, Isabel B. *Some findings with regard to type and manual for Myers-Briggs Type Indicator, Form E.* Swarthmore, Pa.: Author, 1958.

Rexroth, K. My head gets tooken apart. In *Bird in the bush: obvious essays.* New York: New Directions Paperbook, 1959, pp. 65–74.

Russell, W. A., & Jenkins, J. J. The complete Minnesota norms for responses to 100 words from the Kent-Rosanoff Word Association Test. Technical Report No. 11, 1954, University of Minnesota, Contract N8 onr66216, Office of Naval Research.

Spranger, E. *Types of men.* (Trans. by Paul J. W. Pigors). Halle (Saale), Germany: Max Niemeyer, 1928.

Strong, E. K., Jr. *Manual for Strong Vocational Interest Blanks for Men and Women, Revised Blanks (Form M and W)*. Palo Alto, Calif.: Consulting Psychologists Press, 1959.

Terman, L. M. *Concept Mastery Test, Form T manual.* New York: Psychological Corporation, 1956.

Welsh, G. S. *Welsh Figure Preference Test: preliminary manual.* Palo Alto, Calif.: Consulting Psychologists Press, 1959.

Wotton, Henry. *The elements of architecture*. London: John Bill, 1624.

# *Edwin E. Ghiselli* *Managerial Talent*[1]

It is, indeed, an honor for me to have been chosen to participate in this series of annual Walter Van Dyke Bingham Memorial Lectures. It permits me publicly to express my thanks to a man who many years ago gave me guidance in my professional career, and who stimulated my thinking and encouraged my work in industrial psychology. With all of the recognitions he received, and so well deserved, for his many contributions to his profession and to his country, he always remained a warm and understanding man, ever ready to hear out the ideas of others and to foster their development. So today I do not so much feel that I am delivering a lecture, but rather as though I were again spelling out ideas as I did in the past to Dr. Bingham so that they thereby become clearer in my mind.

The University of Michigan is to be congratulated for having been chosen as the site of this lecture. Again recognition is given to this institution, which because of the high quality and quantity of its research and human product, has played, and increasingly

1. This paper is based on the Walter Van Dyke Bingham Lecture given at the University of Michigan, April 26, 1963. It was first published in the *American Psychologist*, 1963, vol. 18, no. 10 (October), pp. 631–642.

continues to play, so unique and important a role in the history of psychology. Yet it is difficult for me to think of the University as an institution since it is peopled with so many friends and former colleagues. So for this reason, too, I feel I am not giving a discourse but rather that I am again taking advantage of the tolerance and understanding of colleagues to talk about some ideas of mine.

As a representative of her husband's profession, I should like to express our thanks to Mrs. Bingham for her generosity in establishing this series of lectures. Throughout his life Dr. Bingham directed his efforts to fostering the full utilization of human resources. He not only saw the value to society of the assessment of human talents, but also its importance for the self-actualization of the individual. By these lectures devoted to the identification and nurture of human talent, his goals continue to be pursued.

Before World War II industrial psychologists largely concerned themselves with the men and women who labor in the factory or keep the books in the office. But in the past 15 years there has been a great surge of interest in examining the nature of those who in business and industrial establishments direct, administer, and organize—that is, manage. I am not at all sure what has caused this shift in interest. I think it not impossible that psychologists have stood in awe of those in high places, viewing managers stereotypically as a category apart from ordinary folk. But now for some reason or another managers are seen as human beings, beings who strive, who bleed, who have feelings, needs, and frustrations, and who differ among themselves in abilities, personality traits, and performances in the same way as do other people. The denizens of Olympus, then, are seen as being of the same stuff as those of Attica.

Psychologists who study management stand accused by critics

of the social scene of a score of trespasses, from surreptitiously destroying individuality among managers to trying to raze the very foundation of American business and industry, individual initiative, with precisely the same objective that brought my great-grandfather to the California mother lode in 1849—gold. And certainly there is some substance for these critics' adverse comments since there has been a plethora of pseudoscientific discourses about the nature and nurture of managers together with a variety of unvalidated action programs for their selection and training. However, much serious work is being conducted, and while our knowledge and understanding is still small, progress is being made in the development of a solid body of empirically determined facts and in sharper and more exact theory. The best testimony of this is the significant work of the social-industrial psychologists here at the University of Michigan, the effects of which are seen throughout the social sciences and in the business and industrial community.

In recent years a group of us at the Institute of Industrial Relations of the University of California—Mason Haire, Lyman Porter, and myself—have been studying the nature of organizations and the psychological characteristics of managers. The investigations of my colleague, Mason Haire (1959), have shown that as business and industrial organizations grow and develop, it is in the very nature of the case that their integrative and coordinative activities assume greater and greater importance. This is indicated by the fact that the larger an organization becomes the greater is the proportion of individuals in it whose functions are of an administrative rather than of a directly productive sort. With the increasing sizes of our business and industrial establishments, then, there would appear to be a real need for psychologists as well as other social scientists to examine the nature of those who manage, so that these establishments can operate as effective organizations.

I shall begin my discussion by trying to define the term manager. I fear my definition will not be as tight as one might wish, but perhaps it will suffice to delineate the general realm of occupational activity wherein I wish to examine talent. Then I shall treat briefly with the problem of gauging success in the performance of managerial activities. I believe that success in management must be viewed broadly, and is not yet readily subject to precise and objective measurement. The main body of my presentation will be concerned with an examination of what I believe to be important facets of managerial talent. In this connection I shall present some of my empirical studies of the psychological properties I have termed management traits. Finally, I shall mention briefly some of our findings on the motives and aspirations of managers, since I believe they will cast additional light on the nature of managerial talent.

While management is reasonably distinguishable as a class in the broad spectrum of occupations, it cannot be said that there is any unanimity of opinion on which particular individuals should be included in it. Perhaps a common root to many of the definitions of the term manager is that a manager is any person in an organization who supervises the activities of others. Such a definition not only includes such first line supervisors as industrial foremen, but also leadmen and craftsmen who direct apprentices, neither of whom are considered to be management personnel. Furthermore, there are some individuals whom almost everyone would place in the category of management, such as safety engineers and legal counselors, who may supervise no one but their secretaries. While certainly one element in the decision of whether to classify an individual as a manager, supervision is not the sole criterion.

Another common root in many definitions of management is that which stems from the meaning of the word to manage. Lexicographically, to manage is to direct, to execute, to carry out, to guide, and to administer, and, interestingly enough, to cope with, to bring about by contriving, and to husband. I am sure that there are many in management who would think that the latter are more descriptive of their activities than are the former. In any event, both arm chair analyses of the job of manager and careful systematic studies of what managers actually do, such as those of Shartle (1956) and the Ohio State University group, give support to the use of functions such as these to distinguish the class of managers in the taxonomy of occupations. Certainly the functions of directing, administering, and the like, do not provide precise criteria for differentiating management positions from those of other sorts, but at least they are guideposts. In general they describe the activities of the persons in the upper portions of the organizational hierarchy.

The personnel of a business or industrial establishment can be roughly classified by level. The individuals at the upper levels are concerned with the overall government of the organization and the formulation of broad plans and policies. Here we find the presidents, vice presidents, and, depending upon the size and nature of the enterprise, those who head major operations or geographical areas. The task of those at the next level is to crystallize the general policies and plans developed at the highest level, formulating them into specific and workable procedures. At this second level are included those who operate divisions or departments in an organization, together with staff personnel who are concerned with specialized activities. The next level are the first line supervisors who are charged with putting into effect the specific procedures prepared at the level above, by the immediate direction of the activities of the line workers. Finally, at the lowest level of the organizational hierarchy are the individuals who directly produce goods and services.

A broad distinction can be drawn between those workers whose activities directly result in the production of goods and services, and those whose activities are of a planful, integrative, and directive character. It is the latter, those in the upper three levels of the organization, who typically are termed management and are distinguished from the producers or line workers. So it is common to speak of three managerial levels, upper management, middle management, and lower management.

If I am to discuss managerial talent, I should, I suppose, be prepared to indicate how a more successful manager can be distinguished from a less successful one. The measurement of job success, the so-called criterion problem, has plagued industrial psychology since its birth. It is not a simple task even with simple jobs, and with management jobs their very complexity makes the problem seem almost insurmountable. The subject has been extensively discussed and empirically examined, but certainly the fundamental issues have not been settled.

Psychologists put great value on precisely quantified and objective appraisals of individuals, appraisals based on concrete and objective measures of each of the various specific aspects of the performance under consideration. While it is obviously true that such appraisals do have many desirable features, I nonetheless believe that there is a case to be made for the purely subjective, global, overall assessments, as are given by one person's opinions or ratings of the performance of another person.

Just because they are expressed in quantified terms, objective measures of performance may erroneously convey the impression that the differences among individuals are great, whereas in fact the differences may be quite small and insignificant. Furthermore, as Likert (1961) has pointed out, those aspects of performance which we can measure objectively, often are quite unimportant and irrelevant. The sharpness with which an executive keeps his pencils can be measured with a high degree of reliability but has little bearing on evaluations of his success as a manager. The relevance and importance of the various activities connected with a job are matters apart from their mode of measurement, and, indeed, are purely value judgments. I do not mean to imply that objective measures of managerial behavior are worthless. Quite the contrary. Recent studies of great ingenuity have been most fruitful of ideas, and have given new insights into the nature of managerial functions (Frederiksen, 1962; Tagiuri, 1961). Nevertheless I do not believe that at the present time they are sufficiently well worked out and tested, and do not give the types of evaluations required.

Psychologists have examined extensively the subjective evaluations, or judgments, of one person by another, and invariably find them wanting. It has been endlessly demonstrated that one man's assessment of the performance of another is influenced by all manner of irrelevant matters. A foreman's ratings of the job proficiency of his subordinates may be in part determined by whether the men are Giant or Dodger fans, and the ratings of the vice presidents made by the president of a company may be biased by whether they prefer Brand X or Brand Y political party. Furthermore, two individuals seldom agree perfectly in their opinion of a third, and when they do collusion is suspected.

Yet, the fact that subjective appraisals of performance are not entirely based on irrelevant matters, and there is some and often considerable agreement among different assessors, is too often forgotten. Furthermore, as Bingham (1939b) so clearly pointed out many years ago, subjective appraisals not only permit a meaningful integration of the individual's performance in the various aspects of his job, but also permit an evaluation in terms of the demands of the setting in which the job occurs. For the present, then, I prefer subjective evaluations of managerial performance.

I have been cavalierly speaking of management as if it were a single job. This is, of course, quite incorrect. The managerial occupation includes a wide variety of positions and the differences among them are great. Managerial jobs range from those with considerable personal authority and responsibility to those which are purely advisory. Some are completely enmeshed in a fabric of interpersonal relationships, whereas others are as lonely as the job of lighthouse keeper. While some demand a professional background, others require no special training. In the work of Hemphill (1960) we have the beginning of an empirically based taxonomy of managerial jobs. But we have so few precise descriptions of managerial jobs and the overlap among them is so great that as a group they appear amorphous. They can be classified into some broad categories such as line and staff, or into functional groups such as production, financial, and sales, but such categories are of the grossest sort.

But I do not see this lack of a clearly defined classification of managerial jobs as a serious problem in the study of managerial talent. It seems to me that one of the characteristics of managers is their movement from one position to another. Furthermore, this movement, often but not always in the form of advancement, is especially characteristic of those of superior talent. There is, then, in a successful manager's career a concatenation of transmigrations among managerial posts which are quite different in character. A person manifests managerial talent not just because he performs well in one given type of position, but because he has the capacity to perform a variety of them well, and the adaptability to change from one activity to another quite different activity.

I have so far tried to make two points, first that it is possible through purely subjective judgment to appraise managerial success, and second that in talking about managerial talent and managerial success we should not just consider an individual's performance on a single job but rather his progress through a series of positions, in other words, his career as a manager.

Over the years I have been called on in one connection or another to assess the managerial talent of a number of men. My appraisals were based entirely on an interview with each man, plus his vita, and very occasionally a conversation with his superior or a colleague. I would like to illustrate my points with four short case descriptions. Two of these men I judged to be of superior managerial talent, and two inferior. The careers of two were entirely in one company and the other two made changes from one establishment to another. All four men were college graduates, having majored either in economics or business administration, and all four were in their middle forties when I saw them. From these four cases I think you will be able to see that it is not at all impossible to gauge the career success of a manager without objective and quantitative measures of his performance.

The first man, after a short and unsuccessful 2 years as a college instructor, took a position in the research and development department of a large organization. After 2 years he became the head of a division in the department, and after 2 more the department chief. His outstanding talents as an analyst brought him to the attention of top management, and with increasing frequency his recommendations were incorporated into the organization's policy. At 35 he became assistant vice president for research and development, and the following year vice president. Here he manifested not only executive ability but also the capacity to influence the board of directors whom top management considered to be far too conservative. The vice president for operations retiring, my man was given his position. The interesting thing is that he was placed in this post purely for storage because he was already marked for the presidency. He had no real feel for operations, and both he and his superiors realized it. By 42 he was executive vice president, and by 45 president. Here we have a career which I believe indisputably is a successful one as a manager.

The second man began his career as a salesman for a small instrument manufacturing company. Because of his aggressiveness as a salesman he was made sales manager, and after 5 more years he was made general manager, and finally president and partner. The company had been experiencing lean times, and it was largely as a result of his efforts, both in promotion and in operations, that it became financially strong. Indeed, its position was so good that a larger company made such a handsome offer the partners could not refuse it. His services then were sought and obtained by a firm of underwriters in a policy-making position involving the purchase and reconstruction of small businesses. Again, a career that clearly is a successful one.

The third man began his career with a brokerage house as an analyst. After 8 years he became the head of the bookkeeping division, and by the time he reached his middle thirties he was made supervisor of the office activities. Here he remained until he was 47. Seeing no further possibility of advancement, and none being promised, he left the company and became a real estate salesman. While, to be sure, in this last job he increased his income, the picture of his career as a manager is quite unimpressive, showing a slow rate of advancement with a final plateau at a lowish level of middle management.

The fourth man began his occupational career with an accounting firm. After some 6 years he was "stolen" by one of the company's clients, to head its accounting division. Later he became the comptroller, but after a few years finding himself unhappy with the responsibility, he quit. He then obtained the position of treasurer with a ferry company in San Francisco, even though the salary was substantially less and he knew it was a dying business. In a couple of years the company dissolved when the ferry route was finally bridged. Out of a job he was back where he began more than 20 years before, seeking employment as an accountant. Here is a career with initial growth and promise, but with a later decline; a career one would not term successful. If his success were measured objectively I suppose the trend would be a quadratic with a negative coefficient. But surely with this, as with the other cases, the subjective assessment is sufficiently precise.

There have been many analyses of the psychological traits important in the performance of managerial functions, together with a substantial number of empirical investigations of the measured traits which distinguish management from line workers, and the measured traits which are related to indices of the success of managers (Harrell, 1961). At the University of California we have tried to obtain some notion of the traits which are of prime importance for managers by comparing the self- and role perceptions of managers at different levels, managers and line workers, and successful and unsuccessful managers (Ghiselli & Barthol, 1956; Porter, 1958, 1959; Porter & Ghiselli, 1957). From the constellations of role and self-perceptions which differentiate these various groups, we have endeavored to develop a picture of the significant managerial traits. Material of this sort lends itself to a variety of interpretations, and it is likely others would interpret our findings in ways somewhat differently than we have. Nevertheless, we do believe our interpretations have some validity inasmuch as we have been able to demonstrate that certain of these patterns of self-perception are related in important ways to the manner in which task-oriented groups govern themselves (Ghiselli & Lodahl, 1958a, 1958b).

From these various analyses I have come to the conclusion that important to managerial success are the traits of intelligence, supervisory ability, initiative, self-assurance, and perceived occupational level. I do not mean to imply that success in management is determined solely by these five traits, for certainly there are many others. Nevertheless, it does seem to me that these particular five traits—intelligence, supervisory ability, initiative, self-assurance, and perceived occupational level—play a key role in managerial functions and therefore are major facets of managerial talent. I should, therefore, like to summarize my work on them (Ghiselli, 1955b, 1956a, 1956b, 1959, 1963a, 1963b).

Let me first consider the trait of intelligence. Today we generally accept the proposition that tests of intelligence measure significant psychological properties of the individual. Yet, we do not seem to worry very much any more about what these specific properties are. I suspect there is a certain amount of battle fatigue as a result of the long and indecisive war we psychologists waged among ourselves during the first 4 decades of the century about the nature of intelligence and the validity of tests proclaimed as measuring it. I doubt if there are very many now who consider intelligence as the single all-important ability that Spearman conceived it to be. Rather we tend to think of intelligence tests as measuring a domain of various cognitive abilities more or less related logically if not psychologically. Intelligence we take to be an important determiner of behavior in those situations involving mental power and problem solving, where the individual is called upon to deal with ideas, abstractions, and concepts.

One of the well-popularized results of the first great mass testing of adults, the measurement of the intelligence of soldiers in the American Army in World War I, was the relationship found between level of occupation and intelligence test scores (Bingham, 1937). It was noted that when soldiers were sorted out into groups in terms of their civilian occupations, those in the so-called higher occupations on the average earned higher scores than those in the lower occupations. Since World War I this relationship between level of occupation and intelligence has been demonstrated a number of times. Men in the professions obtain the highest scores, followed in order by those in managerial, supervisory, and clerical jobs, and finally those in the various industrial jobs show average scores in descending order of skilled, semi-skilled, and unskilled workers.

In all of these investigations there is found a substantial amount of variation in scores among individuals in any one occupational group. Thus some factory workers earn higher scores than those earned by some lawyers. Nevertheless, the relationship between level of occupation and measured intelligence is quite substantial.

The intelligence test scores of persons in management positions fall in the higher ranges of the distribution of scores of the general employed population. Furthermore, it appears that by and large those in lower management have the lowest scores and those in upper management the highest ones. There is quite a substantial difference in intelligence between lower and middle management, but the difference between middle and upper management is small. As a matter of fact, lower management and line workers are about the same in measured intelligence. Industrial foremen are about equal to skilled workers, but office supervisors do seem superior to clerical workers. It is probable that among office supervisors are some young people in trainee positions who are slated for higher management positions. The average intelligence test scores of those who hold positions in the upper and middle levels of management is very high, indeed, and is reported to exceed the scores of about 96% of the population (Harrell, 1961). Over the years I have tested several hundred managers at these levels in a variety of different businesses and industries. Interestingly enough their average score, too, happens to fall at the ninety-sixth percentile.

There is a substantial body of evidence which indicates that there is a relationship between level of occupation and the degree to which job success can be predicted by intelligence test scores (Ghiselli, 1955a). As one moves up the scale of occupations from the unskilled to the upper managerial, one finds not only higher and higher average test scores but also higher and higher correlations between intelligence test scores and job success. Nevertheless, even at the upper two levels of management, the relationship between intelligence test scores and job success is by no means high, and while the reported relationships vary in magnitude from one investigation to another, by and large they are perhaps best described as being moderate.

So one might take the position that the greater the measured amount of intelligence an individual possesses the higher he is likely to rise in the organizational hierarchy, and the greater is the probability he will be a successful manager. But I am not sure that the latter part of this generalization can be accepted without question, at least at the higher levels of test scores. There have been suggestions that at the middle and upper managerial levels there is not a simple one-to-one relationship between intelligence and managerial ability. Rather it would appear that the relationship between intelligence and managerial success may be curvilinear, with not only those managers earning low scores being on the average poorer, but also those earning very high scores.

I have found this to be the case with three groups of managers. The average scores of all of these groups were quite high, as I reported earlier they exceeded the scores of about 96% of the general population. In each group I divided the men into those whose scores fell above this point and those whose scores fell below it. In every group, for the men with the lower scores there was a positive relationship between intelligence and success and for the men with the higher scores the relationship was negative. In other words, for individuals of higher and higher intelligence there is a greater and greater probability they will achieve success as managers until a critical intellectual level is reached. This level is quite high, indeed, but above it individuals with higher and higher scores have less and less chance of being successful managers.

For one of these groups, a group of executives in a financial organization, success was gauged by the higher management of the organization. Without in fact knowing what the scores were, it was the men who earned the highest and the lowest scores whom higher management invited to leave. A second group was comprised of individuals the success of whose managerial careers I appraised. I mentioned earlier the nature of these appraisals and gave some examples. These men were employed in a wide variety of different organizations and held a wide variety of different managerial positions. Yet, the careers of those earning the very highest scores were not as successful as the careers of those who earned somewhat lower scores. The measure of success I used with the third group I think is most interesting and significant. For these men success was gauged solely and entirely in terms of how the individual appraised himself. I asked managers to evaluate their own careers, indicating the degree to which they themselves believed they were successful. These reports were, of course, anonymous. It was both the managers who earned very high and low intelligence test scores who viewed their careers with the greatest misgivings. So there does appear to be some substance to the notion that a curvilinear relationship exists between intelligence and managerial success, with the very very bright, as well as those more poorly endowed, being less likely to be successful than those at intermediate levels.

We have seen that the evidence indicates intelligence to be an important factor in managerial success, and therefore it is one of the facets of managerial talent. Individuals of higher and higher intelligence have greater and greater chances of being successful managers. This relationship holds until a very high level of intelligence is reached, and then there appears to be a brief trend in the opposite direction. Individuals who fall among the top 2 or 3% of the population in intelligence are somewhat less likely to be successful managers than those immediately below them. It is possible that those individuals at the very extreme high levels of capacity to deal with abstract ideas and concepts do not find in managerial activities the intellectual challenge they need.

In recent years, discussions of conditions for effective organizations, particularly those discussions with a so-called human relations orientation, have stressed the importance of leadership. Indeed, the naive student might well suspect that the sole function of management is leadership, with top management leading middle management, middle management leading lower management, and lower management leading line personnel who do all the work. The implication seems to be that if management provided proper leadership, both for itself and for line workers, all organization ills would be cured. While it is unquestionably true that one of the functions of managers is to supervise the activities of those lower in the organization, and that the better supervision management provides the better the organization will function, leadership and the supervision of subordinates is only among the many functions that managers perform.

Still, the life of a business or industrial organization lies in the individuals who people it. If the organization is to function as an effective social entity, its human parts must operate in an integrated fashion. As yet, the most effective integrative machinery our species, Homo so-called sapiens, has been able to develop is an authoritarian hierarchy of individuals, a series of superiors and subordinates, ranging in a business or industrial organization from the president at the top to the line workers at the bottom. Except for the individuals at the top and bottom, each person has two roles, one as the supervised and the other as the supervisor. Each has his activities directed by a superior and in turn directs the activities of subordinates. It is not impossible that in the future social science will provide some quite different type of machinery which more fully utilizes the varieties of human talent and increases individual freedom, creativity, and self-fulfillment. In the meantime, we are stuck with a system wherein ability to supervise the activities of others is a primary matter.

I do not think it appropriate here to enter into a discussion of what constitutes effective supervision. Notions about the nature of good supervision vary widely and are likely to be, if I may say so, contaminated by theoretical notions about leadership, and by social views. It does seem clear that what are good supervisory practices in one situation may be poor in another. For my purposes here I shall simply take good supervision to be that behavior which management, in a given situation, says is good supervision as distinguished from that behavior which management says is poor supervision. In other words, I am again taking ratings, or personal and subjective estimates, as an adequate index of success, in this case as a criterion of supervisory ability. The test I use as a measure of supervisory ability I consider to be a valid measure of this trait since, in widely differing organizations, the scores individuals earn on it are related to the ratings of supervisory ability assigned to them. Therefore, I can perhaps say that by superior supervisory ability I am referring to the effective utilization of whatever supervisory practices are indicated by the particular requirements of the situation.

My findings indicate that there is a relationship between supervisory ability and occupational level just as there is with intelligence and occupational level. As one proceeds up the scale of occupations from line workers through lower and middle management to top management there is a progressive increase in capacity to supervise the activities of others. The difference between lower management and line workers surprisingly enough is small. But there is a considerable superiority of middle management over lower management, and an equally great difference between middle and upper management. In capacity for leadership the higher levels of management are quite superior, and the top level of management is outstanding.

As one might expect, with line workers there is little or no relationship between measured capacity for supervision and job performance. But with managers at all organizational levels I find supervisory ability bears quite a substantial relationship to the evaluations of their performance as managers. Indeed, of all of the five traits I have termed management traits, this seems to be of paramount importance. Furthermore, my investigations indicate that supervisory ability is a somewhat more important determiner of success at the upper management levels than it is at the lower levels, though the differences are not great. Ability to direct the activities of others, then, is a significant aspect of managerial talent, and on the average the higher and higher an individual makes his way in the organizational hierarchy the more qualified is he likely to be as a supervisor, and the more important this ability is to his success as a manager.

Many persons in management who possess quite adequate intellectual and social talents and who are highly motivated, nevertheless are sometimes found wanting by their superiors. They do their work carefully, they exercise good judgment, they are zealous, and they are adept at interpersonal relationships. Yet, there is a certain independence and inventiveness which is missing in their performance. Such people are often described as lacking in the quality termed initiative.

At great length managers deplore and bewail the absence of initiative in their subordinates, though they seem less willing to rejoice in its presence. The importance of initiative is stressed at all organizational levels, yet few have addressed it empirically, much less attempted to measure it. Unquestionably initiative is an elusive and vague trait, and is a complex one involving a variety of dimensions of personality. With far less wisdom than I hope is my wont, I have tried both to define and to measure initiative.

It seems to me that initiative has two aspects. One is motivational and involves the beginning of actions, and the other is cognitive and involves the capacity to note and to discover new means of goal achievement. The first aspect involves the ability to act independently and to initiate actions without stimulation and support from others. The second aspect involves the capacity to see courses of action and implementations that are not readily apparent to others. Both aspects have the property of being self-generative. It does not seem to me that initiative implies a capacity to maintain motivation and sustain goal-oriented activity in the face of frustration. Rather a person who possesses initiative is an inaugurator or originator who opens new fields and conceives of novel ways of doing things.

Very likely the test I use to measure initiative is a chancy thing. Even so, I regard it with a certain satisfaction. It is valid in the sense that scores on it are related to superiors' ratings of initiative. But more than that it differentiates those individuals who say they want a job wherein they can use their initiative from those who disclaim any such desire. If I am correct in viewing initiative as being self-generative, then self-reports, such as these reflecting the way an individual proposes to go about things, are of particular importance.

The relationship I find between measured capacity for initiative and age is an interesting one. With line workers there is a progressive decrease in initiative with increasing age, and past the age of 40 initiative shows a sharp and significant drop. On the other hand, with persons in management positions there is a continuous, though small, increase in initiative with age. This suggests the possibility that being in a situation where initiative is not required kills its expression, and being in a job where there are many and continued opportunities to manifest initiative fosters it.

If initiative is an important aspect of managerial talent it should be related to level of occupation; and, indeed, I find this to be the case. Proceeding from line workers through lower and middle management to upper management there is, on the average, an increase in the measured capacity for initiative. Members of upper management appear to be particularly outstanding in this trait. But at all occupational levels there is a wide range of differences among individuals. Even among the laboring groups there is a substantial number of individuals who possess very high levels of capacity for initiative. The supply of people who are outstanding in initiative is substantial. All that is needed is a situation wherein those who possess it can utilize it.

At the upper two levels of management there is a positive relationship between initiative and job performance. The greater the individual's capacity for initiative the more likely he is to be judged as being a good manager. On the other hand, at the lower levels of management and with line jobs, in general I find either no relationship at all between initiative and evaluations of job performance, or a negative relationship. So while initiative might be rewarded at the higher levels of management, at the lower levels it is likely to be punished.

The fourth trait I consider to be an aspect of managerial talent is self-assurance. By self-assurance I mean the extent to which the individual perceives himself to be effective in dealing with the problems which confront him. There are those persons who see themselves as being sound in judgment and able to cope with almost any situation, whereas other people think of themselves as being slow to grasp things, making many mistakes, and being generally inept. The former stand high in self-assurance, and the latter low.

One thinks of the military commander whose utter self-confidence, an almost arrogant self-confidence, permeates his entire troop, reassuring them that all is and will continue to be well, and so impels them to all manner of brave deeds. Undoubtedly the self-assurance of any superior, military or otherwise, often has this sort of effect upon the performance of his subordinates. While certainly self-assurance is often the fool's way, leading him to tread where wiser men will not go, nevertheless it can be the very instrument which enables the individual to deal with his problems and to make decisions about them so that his performance is effective. Because of his confidence in himself he is willing and eager to meet problems head on. Since in many situations any kind of decisive action is better than none at all, the self-confident individual may well achieve the greater success.

Defining self-assurance as I do permits me to demonstrate the validity of my test of the trait in a very simpleminded way. With unbounded self-assurance I simply show that my test differentiates people who believe themselves to be effective individuals from those who believe themselves to be ineffective. I have found that my test differentiates those students who see themselves as scholars from those who see themselves as dunces, those workmen who describe themselves as highly skilled from those who describe themselves as being of lesser proficiency, and those managers who openly admit their performance is excellent from those who confess theirs is lacking.

As with the other managerial traits, as one proceeds from the lower occupational levels to the higher ones there is a greater and greater amount of self-assurance manifested by the personnel at those various levels. There is a substantial distinction between lower and middle management, but also between middle and upper management. Highly placed executives are outstanding in the confidence they have in themselves.

With line workers there is no relationship between their measured self-assurance and their job success. At all three managerial levels there is some, but quite modest, relationship. So while I would consider self-assurance a facet of managerial talent, it, together with initiative, seems to be of lesser importance than intelligence, supervisory ability, and perceived occupational level.

I come now to the fifth and last of the traits I have taken to be aspects of managerial talent, the trait I call perceived occupational level. Whether rightly or wrongly, for good or for evil, we order occupations, as I have done here, from the unskilled through the semiskilled, skilled, clerical, sales, and lower management jobs, to the upper management jobs and professions. The average scores earned by these occupational groups on a variety of psychological traits order them in this manner, or approximately so, and the order reflects their social desirability, their snob appeal, in our society. So in our thinking we have crystallized the notion of a scale of occupations, and we place individuals on that scale in terms of the occupational level of the job they now hold, the job they have the ability to hold, the job they aspire to, and the like.

The monumental work of E. K. Strong (1943) on occupational interests, work stemming from the early research stimulated by Bingham at the Carnegie Institute of Technology, has, among other things, shown that the patterns of interests of persons at different occupational levels are different. Knowing an individual's interest pattern, then, he can be placed on the scale and be described as having the interests of people in the higher occupations, the middle occupations, or the lower occupations.

Just as individuals differ in their patterns of interests so they also differ in their patterns of self-perceptions. Some persons think of themselves as being honest, cautious, and industrious; others think of themselves as being reliable, inventive, and sociable; and so on. Inasmuch as the patterns of interests of workers at different occupational levels differ, we would expect their self-perceptions also to be different. This I have found to be true. I have developed a test wherein the individual describes himself, and these self-perceptions are different for workers at different occupational levels. So I can locate an individual on the occupational scale by ascertaining the level where workers describe themselves in about the same way as he does.

Occupational-level scales based on such matters as interests and self-perceptions generally are considered to measure something akin to level of aspiration. The individual who is placed high on such a scale is regarded as one who wants the responsibility and prestige associated with higher-level jobs, and believes he has the talents required by them. An individual who is placed low on the scale is one who is content with less by way of rewards and status.

By the very nature of my test of perceived occupational level, line workers on the average fall at the lower ranges of the scale and persons holding upper management positions fall at the top, with lower and middle management being intermediately placed. All of the groups are widely differentiated in terms of perceived occupational level, but the largest difference is between lower and middle management. So it would seem that in terms of the way they perceive themselves, line workers and lower management constitute one family, and middle and upper management constitute another family.

I find the same family division in terms of the relationship between perceived occupational level and job proficiency. At the upper two levels of management the relationship between perceived occupational level and job success is positive, and in general at the lower level of management and with line workers it is negative. That is, at the upper levels of management, the more an individual perceives himself in the same way as do those who are in fact high occupationally, the better his performance is judged to be. With lower management and line workers the situation is just the reverse. The more an individual perceives himself in the same way as those who are high occupationally, the poorer his performance is judged to be.

There seems to be adequate justification, then, for considering perceived occupational level as an aspect of managerial talent. Seeing oneself in the same way as those in upper management do would seem to provide the needed stimulation for the individual to perform in ways which insure his moving up the organizational ladder.

I have traced for you my thinking about what I consider to be some of the major facets of managerial talent. Managerial talent has a heavy intellectual component. It perhaps does not represent the very highest levels of abstract thinking, but it does involve the capacity to see and to develop novel solutions to problems. While not synonymous with leadership, managerial talent does manifest itself in the effective direction of others. Finally, managerial talent implies a willingness to depend on oneself coupled with a self-generated impetus to activity and a striving for, and a willingness to accept, the authority and responsibility which goes with high-level positions in organizations. This suggests that the substratum of managerial talent is individuality, and its corollary, the desire for self-realization through creative activity.

Individuality is a term which has very different connotations for different people. Consequently, when one describes a person as being individualistic, some will take him to be a genius and others will take him to be some kind of a nut. If we are to deal with individuality with scientific impartiality we must define it so that the term carries no emotionally loaded meanings. For purposes of examining it empirically, I have defined individuality as the extent to which a person's pattern of traits is unique, that is, the extent to which it is dissimilar from other patterns which are characteristic of many individuals (Ghiselli, 1960).

Therefore, it is possible to conceive of a dimension of individuality. At the one extreme are those persons whose patterns of traits are very different from those of other people, and at the opposite extreme are persons whose patterns are very much like those of a substantial number of people. Furthermore, we can talk about a person's individuality in a variety of domains of behavior. A person might be very individualistic in his behavior which is job connected, doing things in ways which are novel and different, and at the same time he may be quite nonindividualistic in his social behavior, doing just the things that the large proportion of people do in social intercourse.

With a group of men at the level of middle management, I examined individuality in managerial behavior in relationship to job success (Ghiselli, 1960). My results indicated that the men who displayed the greatest individuality in managerial behavior were in general the ones judged to be the best managers. These findings, of course, are counter to the notion so commonly advanced by social critics today that individuality hinders those who aspire to the higher levels of management. Unquestionably there is some substance to the argument that the way to succeed in business is to conform. Indeed, I can give some supporting instances. But I believe the discussions are clouded by poor definitions of the terms "individuality" and "conformity." Furthermore, I am concerned here with managerial talent and individuality in relation to how the individual does his work, and not to how he behaves with respect to the social milieu of his organization.

Haire, Porter, and I are currently engaged in studying the motivations, goals, and attitudes of managers (Haire, Ghiselli, & Porter, 1963; Porter, 1962, 1963). We have questioned several thousand managers not only in the United States but also in a variety of countries throughout the entire world. Not unexpectedly, we find the effects of cultural differences and that the goals of Japanese and Norwegian managers are not precisely the same, nor are those of Indian and Italian managers. Nevertheless, in one respect we find a high degree of unanimity among managers in all countries and at all levels of management. More than anything else, managers want the opportunity to use their talents to the utmost in their work, to act independently, to realize themselves as individuals. Self-realization and autonomy universally are more important to managers than prestige, social satisfactions, and even security.

So I believe there is some substance for my suggestion that the substratum of managerial talent is individuality and the desire for self-realization through creative activity. It seems to me that this gives flavor and meaning to the picture I drew of the talented manager as one who is well endowed intellectually, gifted with the capacity to direct the efforts of others, self-stimulated to action, confident in his abilities, and striving for a position where he can most fully utilize them.

If it seems I am describing a paragon of all the virtues, let me remind you that I am speaking of talent, which, as Bingham (1939a) put it, is exceptional ability. There are managers and managers, and not all of them manifest high levels of managerial talent. Indeed, the proportion of those who do may not be large. Those of greater managerial talent do their work well and advance in their organizations, and those of lesser managerial talent perform in a pedestrian manner, leave management for other employment commensurate with their particular abilities, or at retirement terminate their careers at low or intermediate managerial levels. Furthermore, I would point out that persons with the properties I have called managerial talent might well be ill fitted for other kinds of activities. The picture I have drawn of a person with managerial talent very likely does not well describe the scientist, the physician, nor the politician. So I am not describing that rare individual who could equally well be king, prelate, or general. Nevertheless, the individual with managerial talent is a gifted person, and an unusual one. Proper use of his gifts will give him the rewards and satisfactions he needs and deserves, and at the same time will maintain the wheels turning in industry and the goods moving in business for the benefit of society as a whole.

## *References*


Bingham, W. V. *Aptitudes and aptitude testing.* New York: Harper, 1937.

Bingham, W. V. Administrative ability, its discovery and development. Pamphlet No. 1, 1939, Society for Personnel Administration, Washington, D.C. (a)

Bingham, W. V. Halo, invalid and valid. *J. appl. Psychol.*, 1939, *23*, 221–228. (b)

Frederiksen, N. Factors in in-basket performance. *Psychol. Monogr.*, 1962, *76* (22, Whole No. 541).

Ghiselli, E. E. The measurement of occupational aptitude. *U. Calif. Publ. Psychol.*, 1955, *8*, 101–216. (a)

Ghiselli, E. E. A scale for the measurement of initiative. *Personnel Psychol.*, 1955, *8*, 157–164. (b)

Ghiselli, E. E. Correlates of initiative. *Personnel Psychol.*, 1956, 9, 311–320. (a)

Ghiselli, E. E. Occupational level measured through self perception. *Personnel Psychol.*, 1956, 9, 169–176. (b)

Ghiselli, E. E. Traits differentiating management personnel. *Personnel Psychol.*, 1959, *12*, 535–544.

Ghiselli, E. E. Individuality as a factor in the success of management personnel. *Personnel Psychol.*, 1960, *13*, 1–10.

Ghiselli, E. E. Intelligence and managerial success. *Psychol. Rep.*, 1963, *12*, 898. (a)

Ghiselli, E. E. The validity of management traits in relation to occupational level. *Personnel Psychol.*, 1963, *16*, 109–113. (b)

Ghiselli, E. E., & Barthol, R. Role perceptions of successful and unsuccessful supervisors. *J. appl. Psychol.*, 1956, *40*, 241–244.

Ghiselli, E. E., & Lodahl, T. M. The evaluation of foremen's performance in relation to the internal characteristics of their work groups. *Personnel Psychol.*, 1958, *11*, 179–187. (a)

Ghiselli, E. E., & Lodahl, T. M. Patterns of managerial traits and group effectiveness. *J. abnorm. soc. Psychol.*, 1958, *57*, 61–66. (b)

Haire, M. Biological models and empirical histories of growth of organizations. In M. Haire (ed.), *Modern organization theory.* New York: Wiley, 1959, pp. 272–306.

Haire, M., Ghiselli, E. E., & Porter, L. W. Cultural patterns in the role of the manager. *Industr. Relat.*, 1963, *2*, 95–117.

Harrell, T. W. *Manager's performance and personality.* Cincinnati, Ohio: South-Western, 1961.

Hemphill, J. K. Dimensions of executive positions. Columbus: Ohio State Univer. Press, 1960. (Bur. Bus. Res. Monogr. No. 98.)

Likert, R. *New patterns of management.* New York: McGraw-Hill, 1961.

Porter, L. W. Differential self-perceptions of management personnel and line workers. *J. appl. Psychol.*, 1958, *42*, 105–108.

Porter, L. W. Self-perceptions of first-level supervisors compared with upper-management personnel and with operative line workers. *J. appl. Psychol.*, 1959, *43*, 183–186.

Porter, L. W. Job attitudes in management: I. Perceived deficiencies in need fulfillment as a function of job level. *J. appl. Psychol.*, 1962, *46*, 375–384.

Porter, L. W. Job attitudes in management: II: Perceived importance of needs as a function of job level. *J. appl. Psychol.*, 1963, *47*, 141–148.

Porter, L. W., & Ghiselli, E. E. The self perceptions of top and middle management personnel. *Personnel Psychol.*, 1957, *10*, 397–406.

Shartle, C. L. *Executive performance and leadership.* Englewood Cliffs, N.J.: Prentice-Hall, 1956.

Strong, E. K. *Vocational interests of men and women.* Stanford, Calif.: Stanford Univer. Press, 1943.

Tagiuri, R. (ed.). *Research needs in executive selection.* Boston: Harvard Univer. Graduate School Business Administration, Division Research, 1961.

# *Norman H. Mackworth* *Originality*[1]

Great care is needed when one is choosing a title for an address of this kind. I heard, for example, about the tragic fate of someone who gave a talk about computers entitled "Artificial Intelligence." His audience claimed that it was too autobiographical. By calling my paper "Originality," I feel I could be running a different kind of risk. There is only one way in which I can claim first-hand experience of originality. I have had the good fortune to meet and work with some of the most original people in the world—on both sides of the Atlantic. This has been and is so rewarding that it is only fitting that I should try to add something to what has been said on the subject.

My 10 distinguished predecessors, granted this very real honor, have covered the ground most thoroughly. Furthermore, seven excellent books have recently been published on the subject (Coler, 1963; Gruber, Terrell, & Wertheimer, 1962; Harper, Anderson, Christensen, & Hunka, 1964; Koestler, 1964; Miller,

1. This paper is based on the Walter Van Dyke Bingham Lecture given at Pennsylvania State University, May 27, 1964. It was first published in the *American Psychologist*, 1965, vol. 20, no. 1 (January), pp. 51–66.

Galanter, & Pribram, 1960; Sayre & Crosson, 1963; Taylor & Barron, 1963). It would be foolish to try to summarize this wealth of material; as an alternative, I shall present some ways of looking at *scientific originality.* I hope that some of these thoughts are sufficiently explicit that they can be tested by experiment or administrative change.

## *Problem Solver and Problem Finder*

### *Solving versus Finding Problems*

Most people are quite clear by now that there are real differences between scientists who are largely solving problems and those who are mainly raising questions. The novelist C. P. Snow (1960) notes these two worlds even within the scientific community. He speaks from considerable experience since he took a large part in the relocation of senior scientists in wartime Britain. He distinguishes between those who are better at solving given problems and those who can formulate new concepts not previously studied. Much more research should now be aimed at understanding the somewhat mysterious ways of these problem finders, although obviously it will be a very long time before the deep insights of a Rutherford are analyzable to any extent (Eve, 1939). A crude yardstick for the stature of successful prophets is the number of years that others have taken to prove that they were indeed right. A Rutherford would score as much as 10 on this scale, since he was sometimes very far ahead of the evidence on atomic structure. Great achievements were also made by Turing who sketched the essentials of digital computers about 10 years before these were actually in existence (Armer, 1963; Green, 1963; Oettinger, 1964).

### *Scientific Inflation*

There are several reasons why the distinction between the problem solver and the problem finder is vital. First of all, problem finding is more important than problem solving. Indeed the greatest contribution that can be made nowadays is to formulate new and testable ideas; the scientist who does not speculate is no scientist at all (Hebb, 1958).

Second, problem finding is so very different from problem solving that further intensive study of simple problem solving is not going to add much to our understanding of originality. The broader cognitive processes have to be tackled in general experimental studies of people who are doing problem finding since this is a much more complex process.

A third reason for studying problem finders is that they undoubtedly form a scientific bottleneck. Problem finders are already scarce, yet they are going to be even more in demand as the years go by. This is due to a plain but startling fact. The rate at which discoveries are made now depends more than ever on the number of people who can *formulate* important research problems.

Scientific progress is no longer determined by the number of people who are good at solving problems because already the supreme problem solvers of our day are machines (Feigenbaum & Feldman, 1963; Greenberger, 1964; Minsky, 1963; Reitman, 1964). The scientist will eventually be freed of even more drudgery by digital computers (Wang, 1963). It is therefore all the more surprising that every branch of science is now being held back because thoughtless engineering has seriously handicapped the widespread introduction of these remarkable techniques. Digital computers have not yet been planned to receive messages from humans. For example, one small change in a program may take a week to introduce. Far too few designers have tried to make it possible to change computer programs quickly. No other devices in the world are quite so badly designed from the point of view of ease of human use.

The great designers of this century will be those who produce computers that readily respond to man's changing thoughts. The automation of science will start when friendly thinking aids replace the present rather distant oracles. This advance, however, may well lead to a most serious scientific inflation. A superabundance of problem-solving techniques could cause a famine of ideas. Once their programs are written, machines are very impressive at solving problems. More can be done in 1 day than in a lifetime of unaided calculations. For example, a program written by Wang recently enabled a digital computer to solve as many as 350 theorems, taken from the first 13 chapters of *Principia Mathematica,* in just under 8½ minutes (Pierce, 1964). Similarly, a problem has been answered in 8 seconds that took the astronomer, Kepler, nearly 2 years to solve.

Machines may eventually also assist in problem finding. Real pioneers such as Licklider (1960) and Minsky (1963), as well as Yntema and Torgerson (1961) have discussed some of the extraordinary benefits (and difficulties) of making digital computers more approachable in the sense of establishing two-way interplay between man and machine. The real excitement is due to begin when the computer regularly comes in at the level of a coauthor; in other words, computers will soon work with men at formulating problems in a give-and-take manner. This implies that the scientist sits at his own private keyboard and operates the machine himself, feeding in first approximations in data form and watching for the results. Hopefully, he will always have a programmer beside him as a safety pilot, since really large and fast computers need an experienced hand if disaster is to be avoided (Newman, 1962). Already such computers are being designed to be employed by many users at remote stations via telephone wires. Existing computers are already fast enough to handle as many as 3,000 such private consoles (McCarthy, 1964). It is therefore not just science fiction to imagine that in a few years every competent basic research man in the United States could have this remarkable facility with his own keyboard in his office.

At first these investigators might well be in a state of fascinated anguish. All this potential problem-solving power will be at their fingertips. For the first time they will have absolute freedom to think. Plans will be tested quickly, and analyzed data will pour back from the machine. Nothing-to-do-but-think may be a mixed blessing when creative ideas do not come fast enough (Licklider, 1964). Later, however, these new and stimulating arrangements may greatly accelerate the whole pace of research because researchers will learn the results of their labors so quickly. Publication could be remarkably stimulating and different. Keyboards could rattle away during the night hours to print out messages from selected colleagues. Eventually, however, this would reduce the invisible college effect noted by Price (1961), because fine words coming in quickly and easily from the wilds could make a good man more detectable.

But escape into the future solves few problems in the present, so we should resume our central theme of human talent. Consider, for example, how Houssay (1961) phrased his views as he received his Nobel Prize.

> The most remarkable piece of research apparatus is the human brain. Some people want to buy every piece of equipment known to science. They believe that with a beautiful building filled with modern equipment they have a first rate research institute. That is a superstition. The great discoveries have been made by men working alone [p. 36].

Although this is the general pattern for present-day research, most people do not realize that by far the most usual way for an original concept to start is in exactly one brain. The individual inventor is often more important than any corporate research by a team of people. The man who found penicillin felt that a team of people was fine when you had something to go on, but when you had nothing to go on, a team was the worst possible way of starting. Jewkes, Sawers, and Stillerman (1961) also make a strong case for the idea that the day of the individual inventor is by no means over. They reached this conclusion after carefully analyzing more than 60 of the main inventions of the twentieth century. They found a tendency for originality to show up in areas quite different from the inventor's own field. For example, the automatic dial telephone was devised by a mortician. The inventor of xerography was a lawyer. The pneumatic tire came from a veterinary surgeon. There are remarkably few scientists in the ranks of the inventor. Specialization may have so cramped their inventive abilities that they hesitate to put forward their ideas beyond their own subjects. A related matter is that important general problems involving many disciplines are sometimes not undertaken for a rather similar reason. Experts are often reluctant even to start to discuss problems in which they cannot see the whole picture for themselves. This is rather surprising because all would agree with Barzun (1964) that the aims of science are to discover a network of facts and make general statements about them.

Problem finders are scarce because this kind of basic thinking is very difficult to undertake. Indeed a good problem is often half a discovery. But there are several other reasons—relating to the streamlining of college procedures—why there are not enough idea men. Current mental tests are biased against problem finders because they inevitably favor the solver. Quite recently it was again emphasized that educational psychologists use examinations and intelligence tests which pick out the efficient verbal reasoners rather than the intuitive observers or constructive thinkers (Burt, 1964). The problem finders that do reach college probably insist on setting their own goals and then may become so spiritedly rebellious that some authorities like MacKinnon (1963) even wonder whether all colleges should even try to seek out the potentially creative. Then again, there is a high wastage during the PhD years, since the solution of given problems may not suit the abilities of the problem finder and such candidates may get lost in the rush of deadlines so characteristic of this time.

Certain specific problems simply do not permit any originality at all. Guilford (1963) has termed this kind of activity convergent thinking. Here the problem solver is quite goalbound, as in the ubiquitous and iniquitous multiple-choice examination. For about 20 years, would-be researchers have learned that one answer rings the bell. Guilford contrasts this convergent thinking with divergent thinking, a classification which resembles the comparison made by Bartlett (1950, 1958) between closed and adventurous thinking.

## *The Nature of Problem Finding*

In research, however, many bells ring out for one success, especially in general investigations. Yet basic research is so very fundamental and buried that most people have never even heard of it. Somehow it seems strange that this quiet partner should be so little understood. The National Science Foundation has repeatedly drawn attention to the great potential interest for the man in the street of this adventurous thinking quite characteristic of basic research. They have defined this activity as a continuing search for new knowledge—guided primarily by an interest in learning more about the ways of nature (NSF, 1961). A less ambitious view was that of Cannon (1945). He said that what the experimenter is really trying to do is to learn whether facts can be established which will be recognized as facts by others and which will support some idea of his own. Highly important attempts are now being made by the National Science Foundation, and others, to keep alive the early curiosity that children so often lose during their school years. The individual scientist usually enjoys a keen sense of adventure and excitement. Indeed, the creative researcher is just as involved in his work as is the poet or the artist (Roe, 1964). This is partly because he has developed the sustaining habit of truth, a somewhat rare quality. Wiener (1954, 1964) and Bronowski (1956) have stressed these aspects and emphasized that the good research man also has a feeling for human dignity which he shares with the vast majority of investigators throughout the world.

Genuine satisfactions also come from the exquisite elegance with which laws can be seen to be condensed into concepts. This is best described by Bronowski (1956) who indicated that "science takes its intellectual coherence and imaginative strength from the concepts at which its laws cross, like knots in a mesh [p. 67]." Such order must usually be discovered by methods discussed by Beveridge (1950), Moles (1957), and Bernard (1961); it does not often display itself simply. In a sense, it must be created. Several studies have noted that disorder does not too greatly dismay original-minded scientists. They like to be able to resolve it. They definitely prefer complexity in test situations. It forms a challenge, just like a complicated case is exciting for the medical man. But details and facts are not nearly so interesting for their own sake as for their meanings and implications (MacKinnon, 1962). Creative individuals have an exceptionally strong need to find order where none appears on the surface. The apparently unclassifiable gains their fascinated attention (Barron,

1963). They merely wish to understand the natural world, whereas the more practical man wishes to control it (Snow, 1964). In his important book on the way of an investigator, Cannon (1945) describes experiences in medical research; he notes that curiosity is the mainspring of his inventive and persistent industry. It is a prime requisite for a career of exploration because without it the researcher is dead. For those who believe in it, the unexpected can happen from time to time.

The real mark of the basic researcher is that the unforeseen problem is a joy and not a curse. Paradoxically, the basic research man is searching for the unexpected. That is what he is doing down there grubbing around the roots of knowledge. He is looking for the problems, and that is what his working life is for—not just to hit the targets, but to find them. In other words, an uncharted hill is not an obstacle; it is a new height to be scaled because it provides a different viewpoint from which innumerable details can be seen in perspective.

More than ever, men are needed to try to define the unexpected problems, whether these are to be found in basic research, in space research, or in air defense. There are human aspects of intelligence which have not yet been touched upon in information-processing models of thinking, although this approach has already proved of real value. Digital computers are seriously inadequate as problem finders. Their silent majesty has this major flaw in that they cannot process the unexpected by themselves. Quite often they can be seen marching their troops off in the wrong direction during the battle of ideas (Neisser, 1963). People, however, do not usually have to have their whole program laid out in advance. Hebb (1958) has emphasized that "the better the idea, the more likely it is to have been extremely vague, inchoate, when experimentation began, and to have become definite only as a *result* of the experiment [p. 464]."

An activity like problem finding would seem to be close to the heart of originality in creative thinking in science. The person builds up a mental model of the likelihood of events. Bruner (1957a, 1957b) has described how an information-processing approach to cognition can be used to describe complex thought processes. In his papers, "On Perceptual Readiness" and "On Going Beyond the Information Given," he has primarily aimed at an understanding of how people build up coding systems that apply beyond the situation in which they were learned. Not only are the stimuli from the environment summarized, but new information can be generated. Perceiving accurately under substandard conditions consists in being able to refer stimulus inputs to appropriate coding systems. Where the information is fragmentary, one reads the missing properties of the stimulus input from the code to which part of the input has been referred. Another important paper is on "Memory Mechanisms and the Theory of Schemata" by Oldfield (1964). This summarizes the early views of Head and Bartlett (1932) on the survival of fragments of experience in schemata and indicates how recall consists in their reconstruction. Oldfield also describes how incoming messages might be summarized for storage as common patterns. Inputs departing from such schemata are stored unsummarized, and dominant details will then act as labels for storage and starting points for recall.

The hallmark of the creative enterprise is that there should be effective surprise because only minds with structured expectancies and interests can distinguish real trends from trivial improbabilities (Berlyne, 1960; Bruner, 1962). The triumph of such a state is that it takes one beyond common ways of experiencing the world; this is why original scientists so often fairly bubble with excitement most days of the year. Stimulating tensions are created even by differences between expected and actual circumstances which seem unbelievably slight to the man in the street. The inventor is also often stimulated to further efforts by no more than the differences between a strong mental image of the ideal version of his intended device and the actual miserable achievements to be seen in his prototype equipment. The more abstract thinker enjoys a similar spur—but now the intensity comes from a mismatch between a mental model of reality and experimental evidence from the real world. Visual images of expected events may be so strong in some biologists that Roe (1964) found they were practically watching mental movies. The mismatch may often be based on the difference between this expected state and the *apparent* actual facts of reality rather than the actual facts, since these can be either wrong, scanty, or late (Forrester, 1964).

The need to change a conceptual framework of ideas is yet another reason why originality is so rarely found. Few people can tolerate the ultimate dilemma: Good scientists have to be careful conservatives and wild radicals almost at the same time. An intellectual framework must be acquired by reading and experiment, and then prudently followed to give a basis from which to detect any significant variations from normality. The real test comes when this faithful framework has to be discarded rather quickly because another set of ideas fits the actual events more closely (Polyani, 1963). Conformity is then the cardinal sin. Good scientists must not only be willing to take risks but they must in fact positively enjoy doing so; indeed they have been termed intelligent, bold introverts (Cattell, 1963; McClelland, 1963). They have also been described as logical, opinionated, impatient, intense, thorough, meticulous, reserved, and clannish by Orth (1959). Creative scientists are also unusually hard working to the extent of appearing almost obsessed with their job. The *one* characteristic all of them have had without exception is an intense devotion to their work. They work nights, weekends, holidays, all of the time (Roe, 1964). A sidelight on the reasons for this endless activity at the frontier has been given by Land, who invented the Polaroid camera (Bello, 1959).

> I find it important to work intensively for long hours when I am beginning to see solutions to a problem. At such times atavistic competences seem to come welling up. You are handling so many variables at a barely conscious level that you can't afford to be interrupted. If you are, it may take a year to cover the same ground you could otherwise in sixty (60) hours [p. 124].

Short-term aims often kill long-term objectives. For example, with reports and studies and telephones to be dealt with every minute, nothing great is accomplished, only small work is done (Houssay, 1961).

At the other end of the scale is the data gatherer—the gleaner as opposed to the guesser. Apart from a series of work samples, the best way to detect the problem solver is to ask him which of five specific but very dissimilar areas he would like to study. Often he may be right in saying that he has no strong preference for any of these very different proposed investigations; he has not structured his experience enough to give even vague guidelines for his thinking.

The drawback of the absence of any relevent conceptual framework can be found in trained scientists when they are working outside their usual fields. This has been well described by Blade (1963) who was quite unable to classify the various types of spruce trees found during a vacation in Maine. Being an amateur botanist, he had no structured system of categories into which he could place the very large number of variations to name them in some meaningful way. It was only after several days that he began to recognize the presence of rules that had escaped him at first. All the possible categories had to be thought out for use in a program in the same way as all the possible moves on a checkerboard have been narrowed down into the rules for checkers or chess (Koestler, 1964).

*The Nature of Problem Solving*

Problem solving is more often found in a practical setting just as problem finding can best be studied in the setting of basic research. But basic research and practical research are inseparably intertwined (Naval Research Advisory Committee, 1959). Indeed they help each other just like the two kinds of blood vessels in the body. There are some useful parallels to be drawn between the gathering of information and the circulation of the blood with its system of outgoing arteries and incoming veins. Outward from the heart go these red and practical arteries always subdividing until they end in the diverging capillary tree. Each of these tiny arterial capillaries, therefore, comes to bear on just one small part of the body. This rather resembles the analytic way in which the red-blooded practical answer is found by constantly narrowing down the search to end up with one highly specific choice. For a time the arterial capillaries are indistinguishable from the venous capillaries. But then inward come the blue and abstract veins, always converging and converging to get to the heart of the matter. This merging and synthesizing process broadly includes more and more of the details flowing in the system. The unifying concepts of basic research are therefore found by a grouping together. This entails guiding wider and wider ranges of details into a few deceptively simple pathways, seldom foreseen, and converging into sweeping blue-sky abstractions.

Something of the nature of the early process that takes place at the start of scientific problem solving has been outlined in an exciting manner by Polyani (1963), who made some valuable points by discussing a problem in astronomy. The question was whether the observed deviations from the theoretical path of a planet showed any real regularity against the background of other variations in the same track which arise from observational errors. Were these perturbations quite random, and, therefore, just background noise? Or did they really consist of a definite signal of some significance? Computers already help to a considerable extent in solving such problems. Particularly relevant here are multiple recording techniques to analyze waveforms in electroretinograms; these can average out random effects and detect regularity beneath the disorder. This is a very simple kind of problem-solving behavior. The variations are being detected by a given classification system based on a clear knowledge beforehand of the only way the stimulus can vary.

Much more complex forms of human problem solving have recently been analyzed by some very successful attempts to write programs for digital computers which will simulate human problem solving. For example, Newell, Shaw, and Simon (1958a, 1958b, 1963a, 1963b) have studied the machine solution of chess problems and mathematical theorems by such means. They have found it quite possible to instruct their computers to adopt shortcuts which people often taken in reaching answers (Newell & Simon, 1961, 1963). Their General Problem Solver, for example, is a program which reasons about ends and means. It is capable of defining ends, seeking means to attain them, and, in the process of so doing, defining new subsidiary ends or subgoals to the original end. By breaking down the problem into subproblems, the solution becomes more flexible. Similarly, the problem has sometimes been simplified by omitting certain details. Alternatively, the solution of an apparently related parallel problem is a help. Another favorite shortcut is to work backwards from the end of the problem to the beginning (Simon, 1964). This work has so far been more successful at simulating human intelligence than in replacing it by a more efficient problem-solving machine (Minsky, 1963). The main contribution has been that these authors have given psychologists a language in which they can be both explicit and comprehensive when expressing their theoretical concepts (Miller *et al.*, 1960). This language may sometimes look rather like Braille to the uninitiated, but at least it is clear and definite. The enormous detail in these programs has also made some of their ideas hard to grasp, but in general this simulation approach does enable ideas to be stated quite definitely and their implications to be thoroughly tested. For example, Newell, Shaw, and Simon have already produced programs for their General Problem Solver such that it is quite impossible to tell from step-by-step verbatim records whether the problem was being solved by a man or by a machine. By such methods they have therefore already achieved very considerable advances in the understanding of problem solving by humans (Hovland, 1964; Miller, 1962, 1964; Reitman, 1964).

### *Some Differences between Problem Solving and Problem Finding*

Computer terminology undoubtedly also helps by expressing the relationships between problem solving and problem finding. These two activities look alike at first sight. Indeed it is true that people are in search of a program or an organized set of mental rules whether they are solving problems or finding them. This similarity has rather misled some into believing that problem solving and finding are more closely related than they really are. Newell, Shaw, and Simon (1958b) have even claimed that:

> Creative activity appears simply to be a special class of problem solving activity characterised by novelty, unconventionality, persistence and difficulty in problem formulation [p. 5].

This definition is much too limited in scope compared with the better and more extensive definition by Sprecher (1959); he emphasized the essential fact that a truly creative contribution generates additional creative activity,

> For example, an important scientific theory provides new solutions to problems hitherto unsolved, new perceptions of problems hitherto unperceived, and new discoveries. This characteristic provides a basis for measurement of levels or degree of creativity. At the bottom of the scale, the creative product simply solves the immediate problem to which it was directed. At the top of the scale, the creative product provides the solution not only to the immediate problem, but also to a wide range of related problems, affects broad areas of thought and activity and may even open up new fields of research or technology or other action or progress . . . [p. 155].

Both these definitions, however, lose sight of the main point that there is an all-important qualitative difference between problem solving and finding. It is clear that *problem solving is a choice between existing programs or sets of mental rules—whereas problem finding is the detection of the need for a new program based on a choice between existing and expected future programs.* It is this consideration of possible new plans and their subsequent construction that accounts for the successful additional outburst of related activity that follows a good problem. This can sometimes even come from discarded programs that proved unsuitable for the initial question. The creative scientist often appears to stumble across new problems. To do this he must start by noting the need for looking at data in a fresh way for a given purpose. The alert problem finder must then be able to produce these changes in his mental coding arrangements. In a sense, he can only do this by devising new mental programs or plans and realizing they are more suitable for relating the facts than the existing mental rules. Quite unexpectedly these new programs may also apply to other problems which can now be tackled for the first time.

In comparing problem solving and finding it is sometimes convenient to describe them side by side as in Table 1.

*Some Research Possibilities on Problem Finding*

Problem finding is difficult for computers because at present they are not self-programed, whereas people can change their own programs completely. Unlike machine programs, people can do this repeatedly without losing valuable experience collected over long periods of time. One of the most fruitful research ideas is believed to be to study how people develop new mental programs or plans without starting afresh each time (Miller *et al.*, 1960). Such investigations would be partly experimental and partly descriptive in nature; they should give some leads on how people grind out general laws from collections of facts, to borrow a gloomy phrase from Charles Darwin, who was himself a champion program changer (Darwin, 1902).

Problem finding in research is essentially the establishment of the need for a new and highly complex mental program. This kind of creative activity is one of the most intricate ways in which humans interact with their environment. Such highly intellectual processes are, therefore, too involved to permit adequate analysis by direct study. Very fortunately, however, it may be feasible to dissect out and follow the formulation of new programs in simpler but related situations. The suggestion is to have experimental studies of the classifying of substandard visual patterns—especially the type of task in which rules would have to be formulated to set up satisfactory coding systems from inputs which are either incomplete or faulty (Bruner, Goodnow, & Austin, 1956).

Table 1. Problem solving and problem finding by humans.

| | Problem solving | Problem finding |
|---|---|---|
| Definition | Problem solving is the selection and use of an existing program from an existing set of programs. | Problem finding is the detection of the need for a new program by comparing existing and expected future programs. |
| Objective | To *choose correctly between existing programs*—in order to select the one program that effectively elicits the required actions from a set of possible responses. | To *choose correctly between existing and expected future programs*—in order to devise new programs and to realize that one or more of these would be more suitable than any of the existing programs in eliciting the required actions. |
| Method | Experiment more than thought minimizes the mismatch between the desired and apparent actual states. | Thought more than experiment minimizes the mismatch between the desired and apparent actual states. |
| Outcome | Success is the discovery of one specific acceptable answer to one well-defined problem. | Success is the discovery of many general questions from many ill-defined problems. |

We need then to know more about simple coding, especially how new coding categories are formulated and selected. This work would resemble the studies on the extent to which, for example, the seven million colors are usually summarized into the usual 20 convenient categories (Bruner, Postman, & Rodrigues, 1951). We also need to learn how input categories can be *changed* to suit the circumstances. The reason is simply that we must understand how the scientist appreciates the need for the formation of a new program. He must obviously do this by relating the customary facts to his existing set of categories; in this way he finds that these are not adequate to cover some new way of looking at the usual evidence. The crux of the experimental approach would therefore be to discover how people set up rules for visual pattern recognition. The more we learn about this rule finding, the closer we shall come to some understanding of the coding procedures and categories involved in research and decision making (Tolcott, Chenzoff, Crittenden, Flores, Frances, Kelley, & Mackworth, 1960).

This new mental program in research thinking is inevitably organized so that the plan forms a related set of instructions arranged in rank order. It would be particularly interesting, therefore, to devise studies in which the test subjects had to develop a filing system for unfamiliar visual shapes without knowing the categories into which these fell. The subjects would, however, know that they were intended to make this into some hierarchical set of categories. Initially, the most suitable test material would be a large unclassified collection of hundreds of individual fingerprints. These would be shown in sets of about 10 prints at a time to ease the burden on immediate memory. The subject would then have to indicate which of these prints seemed to be closely related to one another. The set of 10 prints would then be replaced by another set which would now, however, contain some items previously seen. The fingerprints which were most often linked with others would constantly be fed back by the experimenter and included in the changing sample array so that eventually a row of highly typical fingerprints might be obtained in the display; each such print would be rather unlike the other in some respect. Every subject might well end up with a different row of typical fingerprints because there would clearly be many kinds of rules that could be applied. Note, however, that the subject need not even verbally formulate the rules he was using in building up these groupings by cross-reference. He could point at the items that appeared to belong together without giving any reasons (Fano, 1964). If necessary, however, a stand eye camera could also record the track of his line of sight as it wandered to and fro across the row of prints (Mackworth & Kaplan, 1963). These eye tracks might well be specially interesting since they could automatically register fleeting mismatches eventually corrected on the way to the final decisions (Bartlett, 1958).

By such means (and subsequent verbal report) it would be possible to discover the rules that the subject was developing. This could determine how the decision tree was growing, and how far it resembled various standard classification trees known only to the researcher. The emphasis would be on climbing up the roots of this tree and on working toward a few broad categories away from those early insufferable details. Part of the experimenter's task would be to devise meaningful ways of evaluating the suggested categories. For example, he might try out any such proposed clusters of items by giving the selected typical prints to other subjects to use as group samples: In this way he could find out how effective these were in practice as key items expressing rules for classifying shapes.

A side benefit of this kind of work is that it could help to devise machine pattern-recognition procedures. The limiting factor in the power of machines to recognize patterns is the inability of humans to identify the promising features in patterns that would be indicative in classifying them. Nobody yet really understands how people recognize general visual patterns; therefore, computers still find pattern recognition one of the hardest forms of work because no one knows the instructions that the programs should contain (Neisser, 1963; Sayre & Crosson, 1963).

Ideas for rule-finding studies in humans might well eventually come from machines searching and attempting to discover regularity in data. But computers and their programs are not likely to help very much with this at present. Although computers are usually by no means self-programing, they can already improve an existing program—and it is exciting to see these beginnings of computer learning by experience. For example, the machine recognition of specific hand-printed capital letters has led to programs that found for themselves the features that differentiated the various letters (Selfridge & Neisser, 1963). Computers have also been programed so that the skill with which they played checkers improved more or less continuously, since the machine could learn at each move. Samuel (1963) used a novel approach here in that his program provided two different machine players, Alpha and Beta. In this arrangement, Alpha was the front man who played the humans and Beta was the backroom boy acting as a pacer. Alpha often proposed some improvement after each of these matches. But these suggested changes were only accepted by the program after they had been solemnly checked out during a further intramural game between Alpha and Beta!

We may yet see extensive problem finding by machines. There are some very interesting possibilities that could emerge from this description, by Simon (1960b), of the ideal self-programing form of computer instructions for the next step in this remarkable journey. This would no longer be a highly stereotyped program,

> but a program that makes the system's behavior highly conditional on the task environment, on the task goals and on

> the clues extracted from the environment that indicates whether progress is being made toward these goals. It will be a program that analyzes by some means its own performance, diagnoses its failures and makes changes that enhance its future effectiveness [p. 25].

It is already true that a computer program has conjectured new theorems—or supposed theorems—and set up the subgoal of proving these (Newell, Shaw, & Simon, 1958b). But these new theorems were found by working backward from the goal of proving a related theorem—and how often is an associated goal known? Wang (1963) describes generating 1,000 theorems in 1 hour, and it is also true that IBM computers have formed hypotheses in explicit situations (Kochen, 1961). So far, only people have been able to search amongst poorly defined alternatives for vaguely stated objectives. But we have already learned from Hebb (1958) that this is exactly the kind of situation that leads even experienced research men to some of their best ideas. Nevertheless Simon (1960a) has predicted that, before 1970, computer programs will be able to solve the range of problems that humans can tackle including questions that are not at all well structured. To an increasing extent, computers will write their own programs and they may even be able to formulate some problems. But on the whole, man will still be rather better at undertaking vaguely specified problem finding.

There remains, therefore, only one hope for any androboosters like Neisser (1963), Barzun (1964), and myself. Problem finding will always be difficult for machines (if not downright impossible) when even related end goals or subgoals are absent. Basically it is a rather exacting requirement to have to work back from an unknown point—or to have to simplify the mismatch between present position and an unknown destination. Some might therefore hold the view that problem finding is the last refuge for the unaided brain in science—simply because there are people who have this unusual ability to search for the unexpected. Yet even such problem finders would be wiser to join them (rather than try to beat them). Man remains the senior partner for this purpose even if the association is called man-computer symbiosis.

## *The Individual and the Institute*

### *Research Setting*

But no man is an island, least of all the good investigator. The second part of this talk, therefore, considers the relation between the creative research man and other people. In his youth and later he may well have usually been a minority of one, according to Torrance (1962), Getzels and Jackson (1962), and Hofstadter (1963). Any creative character therefore raises special problems as well as the research questions he asks when he enters the doors of a research organization. It is interesting to try to detect at least some of the essential administrative circumstances that facilitate original ways of thinking. Various long lists of the factors involved have been prepared; the best of these being in Taylor and Barron (1963), and in Coler (1963). But these details may obscure the outstanding fact that, in general, the social and intellectual environment is of much greater importance than the physical surroundings. For example, Orth (1959) has recognized that the optimum climate for industrial research is largely determined by the background of opinion set by the management.

Some architectural design features should be mentioned in passing, however, because these make for an easier relationship with others. The first is a comparatively small matter—simply that good air conditioning may be an essential in certain areas to avoid the disastrous lassitude and irritability so fatal for intellectual activity. The second architectural point is more fundamental. There is a need for accidental discussion and casual communication and this can be contrived by what might be termed arranged meeting spaces. The long row of small separate rooms is great for monks but not for research men. In other words, researchers need togetherness from time to time, almost as much as they need to close the door and spare the mind. When, therefore, six or more such doors open on the same meeting place, it is surprising how much easier it is to have a meeting of the minds that initially results from quite accidental encounters.

### *Formation and Destruction of Ideas*

Now, why should it be important to make such elaborate and somewhat tortuous arrangements to encourage mental encounters between scientists? The answer is simply that original people of this kind have inevitably built up their own very strong framework of ideas which need to be tested (to destruction, if necessary). We have discussed how essential it is to build up such a structure. But these same fixed ideas can be an occupational hazard for even the best of men; they can form a door shut against further thinking rather than a ladder to the stars. Such scientists work from a one-reel program. The near-great develop one unique approach to certain problems and never change that mental program. But the really great are kept genuinely humble; they know they are going to have to change and change and change their approach to almost the same set of ideas over and over again. Perhaps they resemble fine generals who can confidently act on the best guess about an exceedingly chaotic battle. They are able to change the rules of their strategy when suddenly the smoke clears to reveal an apparently slight trend in the tactical situation which makes nonsense of their present approach. What we need from a theory is that it should hold together long enough to lead us to a better one (Hebb, 1958).

Frequent meetings with others are therefore vital, a matter considered by Hughes (1963) in some detail. Original people have inevitably built up such a rigid structure of ideas that it takes a head-on collision with an equally strong (or even more rigid) mental structure of a different kind to have the desired effect. This effect will be to convert that endless journey round one single skull into more than the regular creaking of a mental treadmill. The more eminent the skull, the further it has to travel to find the few people in the world who can put these revered but imprisoned brains into new and better shape. Henle (1962) interestingly discusses the need to consider the death of old ideas as well as the birth of new concepts.

The painless way of altering research assumptions is the well-known working-research fellowship, lasting perhaps a year. This can blur the stored mental patterns sufficiently to permit a recombining of their elements into quite new shapes. I was privileged to help Sir Frederic Bartlett start a series of such visits from the United States to the Medical Research Council's Applied Research Unit in Cambridge, England. My successor there, Donald Broadbent, has done such a fine job that a whole series of National Science Foundation fellowships has been held there in the last few years. The host unit also greatly benefits by such visits, and I believe the advantages of this idea could be extended if in general the host institute in England could provide a nucleus of workers to be associated with the visitor in some new field. They can then continue the good work when the visitor returns to the United States.

There is another administrative experiment which is currently in progress at many universities. This is the establishment of multidisciplinary research centers which are able to provide opportunities to meet specialists from other fields. I believe that such institutes can do a great deal of good to provide stimulating research surroundings in university settings. In the Harvard Center of Aerospace Health and Safety, for example, Ross McFarland has brought together medical men and engineers, psychologists, physiologists, and anthropologists. Similarly in the Harvard Center for Cognitive Studies, Jerome Bruner and George Miller have associated psychologists, sociologists, physiologists, computer experts, mathematicians, linguists, and philosophers. The success of such arrangements undoubtedly depends on the feeling of common purpose that can be developed so that the various individuals work together really effectively. Hebb (1958) mentions the stimulation to new ideas, the criticism and guidance that is possible when workers with different backgrounds and skills effectively understand one another's languages and modes of thought. This genuine cooperation is characterized mainly by people exchanging ideas before and during the experimental phase of their investigations rather than after their work has been completed. A suggestion here is to encourage people to have at least two research problems. One would be their own individual work which would occupy most of their time. The other problem would, however, be a group research study, perhaps 1 day a week. Groups of not more than six scientists would meet on common ground over a shared topic of investigation conducted on the same research subjects or patients.

One of the most successful experiments of this cooperative type is to be found in the University of California's San Francisco Medical Center, where there is the Cardiovascular Research Institute, directed by Julius Comroe, also the Professor of Physiology. It is interesting that this group received a 7-year grant in 1961 from the Public Health Service. They mention in the 1961–62 annual report from the Institute that this long-term support has many advantages (Comroe, 1962).

> It provides stable support for many competent scientists for whom there are no university-supported positions. It permits individual scientists to spend more time in research than in grant administration. It encourages long-term research planning and an attack on difficult, long-term problems rather than on easier problems which provide quick answers [p. 14].

*Research Support*

It would be logical for this trend towards longer-term grants to continue, as the Government's own Office of Naval Research maintains that basic research is indeed a long-term affair with them since the average length of their projects was 5 years in 1959. The National Science Foundation has also taken the lead by publishing recently a report entitled "Investing in Scientific Progress," which has many useful ideas on the scientific and educational requirements during the present decade (NSF, 1961).

Some outstandingly interesting comments have been made by Roth (1963). He speaks as a Special Assistant to the National Aeronautics and Space Administration; he is able to indicate the general educational reforms required, since he is also Professor of Mathematics at New York University. Then, as Director of the Office of Research Services, he goes on to specify 10 important ideas on educational research. Roth suggests, for example, that bright students (both undergraduate and graduate) who are believed to be potentially creative might be permitted to forgo formal classwork in their major fields to enable them to work under the supervision of a keen faculty member. He favors the use of institutional grants to universities rather than a reliance on grants and contracts awarded to individuals. On the other hand, the National Institutes of Health have found a way of supporting individual scientists by career awards through universities. This arrangement has one great merit for Government and investigator alike; it encourages the open and free discussion of research ideas and plans. Direct support of separate research projects often stifles such discussions before the ideas are sold to the Government.

At the risk of being thought to be against motherhood, I want to mention the hypothetical case of the $30,000 contract for 1 year. Let us suppose that each of 30 groups throughout the country spend $1,000 on proposal writing and travel to meetings to try to win such support. Then, across the country as a whole, the actual cost of writing such proposals would seem to amount to the value of the contract itself. Not all the unsuccessful efforts would be lost by any means, since proposal writing and evaluating are forms of problem finding. But it is hard to follow the economics of it, despite the obvious benefits resulting from competition between groups of people rather than between individuals.

Land (1964) has recently discussed (in one of his all too rare publications) the various dilemmas facing any government that would like to support inventions. He indicates that government support is not likely to be forthcoming for inventions because government funds are liable to be kept for ventures that usually succeed—and most inventions fail financially.

The balance between stability and change has to be held within society as well as within the investigator:

> Invention involves breaking through a series of barriers which are both intellectual and social. . . . Nearly every worthwhile invention will thus seem to be a war comprising many battles, every battle being against fixed attitudes. These fixed attitudes are fundamental human characteristics that are of the very nature of life and society. Our survival from moment to moment depends upon them. . . . The paradoxical problem which society must face is that on the one hand its stability depends on resisting change but its growth, vitality and healthy future depend on the cautious substitution of

> new arrays of order for old arrays of order. . . . How can we protect an individual from the group when an individual is seeking to destroy a sequential array of attitudes and replace them with a new sequence which in his opinion will be better for society? . . . Rigidity is the other name for people in the aggregate. . . . Society cannot know novelty because it is rigid and yet it proposes to protect and affirm the novelty of what the inventor offers. Yet the patent system protects and encourages the inventor and makes possible the long, long investment by his associates in the most exciting and fantastic kind of gamble there is: a gamble not for the victory of a horse but a gamble for the grand victory of some great new contribution to our society [p. 159].

But the fact that perhaps less than 1 invention in 50 makes any money at all is in some ways all to the good. Financial disasters can emphasize the lasting advantages of intellectual activity. In his new book entitled *From Dream to Discovery,* Selye (1964) remarks that his father twice lost all his possessions and then told his son, who eventually achieved fame as a biochemist, that studying and research gave possessions that could never be lost. There are other satisfactions, too. Our century has seen one of the greatest investigators of all time, Sir Alexander Fleming. He once laughed along in a talk to some medical students in Cambridge, England, that he had heard from friends that a certain amount of money was being made out of penicillin. In fact, his achievement was measured in somewhat different terms—because he knew he had saved more lives by this discovery than any one man ever had before in the whole human history (Maurois, 1959). Although Sir Alexander Fleming was also a Scotsman, I must admit that Scotland has had no monopoly on great men.

*Only One Brain*

Let me mention, for example, one of the finest scientists that the United States has ever had—Robert Goddard. Even he found it difficult to gain a hearing, at first. As early as 1910, he wrote a paper on the "Possibility of Navigating Interplanetary Space." But this was obviously such a wild and really far-out idea that a popular scientific journal turned it down.

Now that the United States has 20-billion-dollar plans to reach the moon, it is interesting to record that these efforts, costing about 10 million dollars a day, started with this very same wild dream. Goddard himself realized it would be the last pioneering expedition to be made by humans (Dewey, 1962). It was exactly 50 years ago this summer that the principles of modern rockets were clearly established when Goddard was granted the first patents on a multistage rocket in 1914. There were all the essential rocket features such as, (*a*) the combustion chamber with its nozzle, (*b*) the system of feeding fuel, and (*c*) the multistage idea. They constituted the fruits of one man's work at research. The discoveries had all been made but were expressed in miniature. Goddard's little rocket was about a foot long and weighed only a few pounds. Then several thousands of men got to work, and 50 years later on January 19, 1964, the Saturn I rocket roared skywards. This successful monster was now more than 200 feet long and many tons in weight. These further changes that produced the largest rocket in the world were the result of development as opposed to research activities. One man did the early research and then tens of thousands of people followed through with the development. These magnificent further technical achievements by Wernher von Braun and his team, among others, led to widespread congratulations for a fine group who had obviously done really important work. But who remembered

Goddard, the man who had sparked off this whole idea? This answer is contained in the following story of the two hats. During the celebrations, President Johnson joked that von Braun might now have some difficulty in fitting on the hat he had recently been given in Texas. But there was no mention of the other hat, that battered, old straw hat Goddard used to wear during all those long years of field trials. For 2 years Goddard had deliberately left this hat gathering dust on the empty laboratory bench when he had to close down his laboratory between the wars due to lack of government funds. This straw hat was a sign that he would return—which he did. But few seem to remember him at all nowadays.

## *Conclusions*

Let me end on a note of cautious optimism. I believe Walter Van Dyke Bingham had a farseeing idea when he proposed these lectures on the "Discovery and Development of Exceptional Abilities and Capabilities." His concern was to help the individual and his feeling for human dignity was what placed Bingham himself in a very special category. Surely we can now look forward with some real hope that talent will not always pass unrecognized. Very many examples could be given, but let me mention only three great Americans whose talents have done so much for psychology. Their achievements have demonstrated that the present situation as regards talent discovery and development can indeed work remarkably well at times. I think of Walter Miles, Henry Imus, and Norbert Wiener—a great research man, a great administrator, and a great thinker, respectively. These three kinds of talents have been brought to bear on some of the hardest problems of our age. Surely no system is too far wrong if such men can reach the top? You all know how Walter Miles has epitomized the ingenuity of the experimentalist. Similarly,

Henry Imus stands as a fine executive with a flair for supporting good research men. Norbert Wiener has demonstrated the deep originality of the thinker. It was a great friend of Wiener's, Sir Frederic Bartlett (1958), who noted in his book on *Thinking, an Experimental and Social Study* that the most important feature of original experimental thinking was the discovery of overlap and agreement where formerly only isolation and difference were recognized. This was certainly characteristic of Wiener who crossed so many boundaries, both national and scientific. As a scientific tribute let me say that the first part of my summary is based on one of his last talks at Massachusetts Institute of Technology (Wiener, 1964).

*Summary*

1. Originality and individuality are badly needed in science—more than ever before.

2. The current information explosion is not at all what it seems to be; more bad papers only make it harder to find the good ones. "Keep the monkeys away from the typewriters!" (This cogent cry from Wiener ranks with Rutherford's delightful dictum: "Go home, my boy— and think!")

3. Intellectual honesty is also required in the sense of willingness to take a chance on the tougher problems as well as on the easier ones.

4. Make some mistakes and admit them. More promising problems may be found in the ruins of these failures. "It is better to be naive and productive, than sophisticated, hypercritical and sterile [Hebb, 1958, p. 464]."

5. Since unifying statements rather than detailed facts are the ultimate general aim, experimentalists should speculate in print more then they do on the broad implications of their work; this may lead on to even more meaningful questions.

6. There is no more fascinating problem in the world than the study of the kind of people who do scientific research. Take heart, however, if their activities are not yet all quite clear. We are ourselves setting out on the long pilgrimage involved in every creative venture. This has been ably defined (Roe, 1963) as "a way of life which emerges from a background of absorption in a topic and begins in a state of imaginative, muddled suspense [p. 177]."

7. Finally, it was John F. Kennedy who said so briefly that one man can make a difference and that every man should try.

### *References*

Armer, P. Attitudes toward intelligent machines. (Orig. publ. 1960.) In E. A. Feigenbaum & J. Feldman (eds.), *Computers and thought.* New York: McGraw-Hill, 1963.

Barron, F. The needs for order and for disorder as motives in creative activity. In C. W. Taylor & F. Barron (eds.), *Scientific creativity: Its recognition and development.* New York: Wiley, 1963.

Bartlett, F. C. *Remembering.* Cambridge: Cambridge Univer. Press, 1932.

Bartlett, F. C. Programme for experiments on thinking. *Quarterly Journal of Experimental Psychology,* 1950, 145–162.

Bartlett, F. C. *Thinking, an experimental and social study.* London: Allen & Unwin, 1958.

Barzun, J. *Science: the glorious entertainment.* New York: Harper & Row, 1964.

Bello, F. The magic that made Polaroid. *Fortune,* 1959, 59, 124–129.

Berlyne, D. E. *Conflict, arousal, and curiosity.* New York: McGraw-Hill, 1960.

Bernard, Claude. *An introduction to the study of experimental medicine.* (Orig. publ. 1865.) New York: Collier Books, 1961.

Beveridge, W. I. B. *The art of scientific investigation.* London. Heinemann, 1950.

Blade, E. Creative science. In M. A. Coler (ed.), *Essays on creativity in the sciences.* New York: New York Univer. Press, 1963.

Bronowski, J. *Science and human values.* New York: Harper, 1956.

Bruner, J. S. On going beyond the information given. In *Contemporary approaches to cognition.* Cambridge: Harvard Univer. Press, 1957. (Reprinted in R. J. C. Harper, C. C. Anderson, C. M. Christensen, & S. M. Hunka (eds.), *The cognitive processes: readings.* Englewood Cliffs, N.J.: Prentice-Hall, 1964.) (a)

Bruner, J. S. On perceptual readiness. *Psychological Review,* 1957, *64,* 123–152. (Reprinted in R. J. C. Harper, C. C. Anderson, C. M. Christensen, & S. M. Hunka (eds.), *The cognitive processes: readings.* Englewood Cliffs, N.J.: Prentice-Hall, 1964.) (b)

Bruner, J. S. The conditions of creativity. (Orig. publ. 1958.) In H. E. Gruber, G. Terrel, & M. Wertheimer (eds.), *Contemporary approaches to creative thinking,* New York: Atherton Press, 1962.

Bruner, J. S., Goodnow, J. J., & Austin, G. A. *A study of thinking.* New York: Wiley, 1956.

Bruner, J. S., Postman, L., & Rodrigues, J. Expectation and the perception of color. *American Journal of Psychology,* 1951, *64,* 216–227.

Burt, C. Foreword in A. Koestler, *The act of creation.* New York: Macmillan, 1964.

Cannon, W. *The way of an investigator.* New York: Norton, 1945.

Cattell, R. B. The personality and motivation of the researcher from measurements of contemporaries and from biography. In C. W. Taylor & F. Barron (eds.), *Scientific creativity: its recognition and development.* New York: Wiley, 1963.

Coler, M. A. (ed.). *Essays on creativity in the sciences.* New York: New York Univer. Press, 1963.

Comroe, J. The 1961–1962 annual report, 1962, University of California, Cardiovascular Research Institute, San Francisco Medical Center.

Darwin, F. (ed.). *Charles Darwin.* London: Murray, 1902.

Dewey, A. P. *Robert Goddard, space pioneer.* Boston: Little, Brown, 1962.

Eve, A. S. *Rutherford.* New York: Macmillan, 1939.

Fano, R. M. Discussion of a library for 2000 A.D. (Orig. publ. 1961.) In M. Greenberger (ed.), *Computers and the world of the future.* Cambridge: M.I.T. Press, 1964.

Feigenbaum, E. A., & Feldman, J. (eds.). *Computers and thought.* New York: McGraw-Hill, 1963.

Forrester, J. W. Managerial decision making. (Orig. publ. 1961.) In M. Greenberger (ed.), *Computers and the world of the future.* Cambridge: M.I.T. Press, 1964.

Getzels, J. W., & Jackson, P. W. *Creativity and intelligence.* New York: Wiley, 1962.

Green, B. F. *Digital computers in research.* New York: McGraw-Hill, 1963.

Greenberger, M. (ed.). *Computers and the world of the future.* Cambridge: M.I.T. Press, 1964.

Gruber, H. E., Terrell, G., & Wertheimer, M. (eds.). *Contemporary approaches to creative thinking.* New York: Atherton Press, 1962.

Guilford, J. P. Intellectual resources and their values as seen by scientists. In C. W. Taylor & F. Barron (eds.), *Scientific creativity: its recognition and development.* New York: Wiley, 1963.

Harper, R. J. C., Anderson, C. C., Christensen, C. M., & Hunka, S. M. (eds.). *The cognitive processes: readings.* Englewood Cliffs, N. J.: Prentice-Hall, 1964.

Hebb, D. O. Alice in Wonderland or psychology among the biological sciences. In H. F. Harlow & C. N. Woolsey (eds.), *Biological and biochemical bases of behavior.* Madison: Univer. Wisconsin Press, 1958.

Henle, Mary. The birth and death of ideas. In H. E. Gruber, G. Terrell, & M. Wertheimer (eds.), *Contemporary approaches to creative thinking.* New York: Atherton Press, 1962.

Hofstadter, R. *Anti-intellectualism in American life.* New York: Knopf, 1963.

Houssay, B. My struggle for science. *World Health,* 1961, Sept.–Oct., 36.

Hovland, C. I. Computer simulation of thinking. (Orig. publ. 1960.) In R. J. C. Harper, C. C. Anderson, C. M. Christensen, & S. M. Hunka (eds.), *The cognitive processes: readings.* Englewood Cliffs, N. J.: Prentice-Hall, 1964.

Hughes, H. K. Individual and group creativity in science. In M. A. Coler (ed.), *Essays on creativity in the sciences.* New York: New York Univer. Press, 1963.

Jewkes, J., Sawers, D., & Stillerman, R. *The sources of invention.* London: Macmillan, 1961.

Kochen, M. Experimental study of "hypothesis formation" by computer. In C. Cherry (ed.), *Information theory fourth London symposium.* London: Butterworths, 1961.

Koestler, A. *The act of creation.* New York: Macmillan, 1964.

Land, E. The role of invention in organized society. *Product Engineering,* 1964, March 2, 159.

Licklider, J. C. R. Man-computer symbiosis. *IRE Transactions on Human Factors in Electronics,* 1960, *1,* 4–11.

Licklider, J. C. R. Discussion on the computer in the university. (Orig. publ. 1961.) In M. Greenberger (ed.), *Computers and the world of the future.* Cambridge: M.I.T. Press, 1964.

McCarthy, J. Time-sharing computer systems. (Orig. publ. 1961.) In M. Greenberger (ed.), *Computers and the world of the future.* Cambridge: M.I.T. Press, 1964.

McClelland, D. C. The calculated risk: an aspect of scientific performance. In C. W. Taylor & F. Barron (eds.), *Scientific creativity: its recognition and development.* New York: Wiley, 1963.

MacKinnon, D. W. The personality correlates of creativity: a study of American architects. In G. S. Nielsen (ed.), *Proceedings of the XIV International Congress of Applied Psychology, Copenhagen, 1961.* Vol. 2. Copenhagen: Munksgaard, 1962, pp. 11–39.

MacKinnon, D. W. Measurement of creativity. Unpublished manuscript, Harvard College Admissions Institute, July 1963.

Mackworth, N. H., & Kaplan, I. Points of view and lines of sight. *Ikon,* 1963, *13,* 45–60.

Maurois, A. *The life of Sir Alexander Fleming.* New York: Dutton, 1959.

Miller, G. A. The study of intelligent behavior. (Orig. publ. 1961.) In A. Oettinger (ed.), *Proceedings of a Harvard symposium on digital computers and their applications.* Cambridge: Harvard Univer. Press, 1962.

Miller, G. A. (ed.). *Mathematics and psychology.* New York: Wiley, 1964.

Miller, G. A., Galanter, E., & Pribram, K. H. *Plans and the structure of behavior.* New York: Holt, Rinehart & Winston, 1960.

Minsky, M. Steps towards artificial intelligence. (Orig. publ. 1961.) In E. A. Feigenbaum & J. Feldman (eds.), *Computers and thought.* New York: McGraw-Hill, 1963.

Moles, A. A. *La création scientifique.* Genève: René Kister, 1957.

National Science Foundation. *Investing in scientific progress.* Washington, D.C.: NSF, 1961.
Naval Research Advisory Committee. *Basic research in the Navy.* Washington, D.C.: United States Department of Commerce, Office of Technical Services, 1959.
Neisser, U. The imitation of man by machine. *Science,* 1963, *139,* 193–197.
Newell, A., Shaw, J. C., & Simon, H. Elements of a theory of human problem solving. *Psychological Review,* 1958, *65,* 151–166. (a)
Newell, A., Shaw, J. C., & Simon, H. The processes of creative thinking. Report No. P-1320, 1958, Rand Corporation. (b)
Newell, A., Shaw, J. C., & Simon, H. Chess playing programs and the problem of complexity. (Orig. publ. 1958.) In E. A. Feigenbaum & J. Feldman (eds.), *Computers and thought.* New York: McGraw-Hill, 1963. (a)
Newell, A., Shaw, J. C., & Simon, H. Empirical explorations with the logic theory machine: A case study in heuristics. (Orig. publ. 1957.) In E. A. Feigenbaum & J. Feldman (eds.), *Computers and thought.* New York: McGraw-Hill, 1963. (b)
Newell, A., & Simon, H. A. Computer simulation of human thinking: *Science,* 1961, *134,* 2011–2017.
Newell, A., & Simon, H. GPS, a program that simulates human thought. (Orig. publ. 1961.) In E. A. Feigenbaum & J. Feldman (eds.), *Computers and thought.* New York: McGraw-Hill, 1963.
Newman, E. B. Paracomputers in psychological research. (Orig. publ. 1961.) In A. Oettinger (ed.), *Proceedings of a Harvard symposium on digital computers and their applications.* Cambridge: Harvard Univer. Press, 1962.
Oettinger, A. G. Programming the Edsac to go shopping. (Orig. publ. 1952.) In G. A. Miller (ed.), *Mathematics and psychology.* New York: Wiley, 1964.
Oldfield, R. C. Memory mechanisms and the theory of schemata. (Orig. publ. 1954.) In R. J. C. Harper, C. C. Anderson, C. M. Christensen, & S. M. Hunka (eds.), *The cognitive processes: readings.* Englewood Cliffs, N.J.: Prentice-Hall, 1964.
Orth, C. D. The optimum climate for industrial research. *Harvard Business Review,* 1959, *37,* 55–64.
Pierce, J. R. What computers should be doing. (Orig. publ. 1961.) In

M. Greenberger (ed.), *Computers and the world of the future.* Cambridge: M.I.T. Press, 1964.

Polyani, M. Experience and the perception of pattern. In K. M. Sayre & F. J. Crosson, *The modeling of mind: computers and intelligence.* Notre Dame: Univer. Notre Dame Press, 1963.

Price, D. J. de S. *Science since Bablyon.* New Haven: Yale Univer. Press, 1961.

Reitman, W. R. Information-processing models in psychology. *Science,* 1964, *144,* 1192–1198.

Roe, Anne. Psychological approaches to creativity in science. In M. A. Coler (ed.), *Essays on creativity in the sciences.* New York: New York Univer. Press, 1963.

Roe, Anne. *The making of a scientist.* New York: Dodd, Mead, 1964.

Roth, S. G. Creativity in an academic atmosphere. In M. A. Coler (ed.), *Essays on creativity in the sciences.* New York: New York Univer. Press, 1963.

Samuel, A. L. Some studies in machine learning using the game of checkers. (Orig. publ. 1959.) In E. A. Feigenbaum & J. Feldman (eds.), *Computers and thought.* New York: McGraw-Hill, 1963.

Sayre, K. M., & Crosson, F. J. *The modeling of mind: computers and intelligence.* Notre Dame: Univer. Notre Dame Press, 1963.

Selfridge, O., & Neisser, U. Pattern recognition by machine. (Orig. publ. 1960.) In E. A. Feigenbaum & J. Feldman (eds.), *Computers and thought.* New York: McGraw-Hill, 1963.

Selye, Hans. *From dream to discovery.* New York: McGraw-Hill, 1964.

Simon, H. A. The corporation: will it be managed by machines? In M. Anshen & G. L. Bach (eds.), *Management and corporations, 1985.* New York: McGraw-Hill, 1960. (a)

Simon, H. A. *The new science of management decision.* New York: Harper & Row, 1960. (b)

Simon, H. A. Simulation of human thinking. (Orig. publ. 1961.) In M. Greenberger (ed.), *Computers and the world of the future.* Cambridge: M.I.T. Press, 1964.

Snow, C. P. *The search.* New York: Signet, 1960.

Snow, C.P. *The two cultures: and a second look.* New York: Mentor, 1964.

Sprecher, T. B. Chairman's report on criteria of creativity at Third Utah Conference, 1959. Cited by Anne Roe in Psychological approaches to creativity in science, in M. A. Coler (ed.), *Essays on creativity in the sciences.* New York: Univer. Press, 1963, p. 155.

Taylor, C. W., & Barron, F. (eds.). *Scientific creativity: its recognition and development.* (National Science Foundation Utah Conferences, 1955, 1957, 1959) New York: Wiley, 1963.

Tolcott, M., Chenzoff, A. P., Crittenden, R. M., Flores, I., Frances, A. S., Kelley, C. R., & Mackworth, N. H. Human decision making as related to air surveillance systems. *United States Air Force Command and Control Division Technical Report,* 1960, No. 61–9.

Torrance, E. P. *Guiding creative talent.* Englewood Cliffs, N.J.: Prentice-Hall, 1962.

Wang, H. Towards mechanical mathematics. (Orig. publ. 1960.) In K. M. Sayre & F. J. Crosson (eds.), *The modeling of mind: computers and intelligence.* Notre Dame: Univer. Notre Dame Press, 1963.

Wiener, N. *The human use of human beings: cybernetics and society.* Garden City, N.Y.: Doubleday, 1954.

Wiener, N. Intellectual honesty and the contemporary scientist. *M.I.T. Technology Review,* 1964, *66,* 17–18, 44–47.

Yntema, D. B., & Torgerson, W. S. Man-computer cooperation in decisions requiring common sense. *IRE Transactions on Human Factors in Electronics,* 1961, *2,* 20–26.

*Philip E. Vernon*

# *Ability Factors and Environmental Influences*[1]

I am deeply appreciative of the honor of being invited to give this year's Walter Van Dyke Bingham Lecture, and would especially like to applaud the initiative of Mrs. Bingham and the American Psychological Association Committee in including some psychologists from outside the United States in their scheme. England indeed has been greatly favored by the selection first of Cyril Burt, then of Norman Mackworth and myself; and I think that this is appropriate, because the Binghams had many friends and were widely respected among British applied psychologists. But might I venture to suggest that the Committee will also sometimes look further afield and consider whether other suitable lecturers might not be found, perhaps from France or Scandinavia, perhaps Canada or Australia? I would like also to take this opportunity to express my thanks to the Local Committee, and particularly to Robert Perloff, for the efficiency and the generosity of their arrangements. It is a special pleasure to visit Purdue University, which has long been associated in my

1. This paper is based on the Walter Van Dyke Bingham Lecture given at Purdue University, April 21, 1965. It was first published in the *American Psychologist*, 1965, vol. 20, no. 9 (September), pp. 723–733.

mind with contributions to applied psychology, for example with the work of Joseph Tiffin, Hermann Remmers, and Charles Lawshe.

Although I have not, like some previous lecturers, had the privilege of close professional contacts with Dr. Bingham, apart from friendly meetings at International Congresses, I have always admired *Aptitudes and Aptitude Testing* (Bingham, 1937) as one of the most sound and comprehensive treatments of the topic. During World War II it was a main textbook for the British military psychologists and personnel selection officers whom we trained for allocation of recruits to suitable trades. Bingham and Moore's (1931) *How to Interview* is likewise still a valuable text for occupational psychologists. And on looking up Dr. Bingham's career, I was delighted to find that his first love was the psychology of music and that he eventually came to vocational and military testing via educational psychology, for these are the areas in which I too have chiefly been interested.

In *Aptitudes and Aptitude Testing*, Walter Van Dyke Bingham (1937) clearly attaches major importance to general intelligence, as I wish to do today. But he took no doctrinaire theoretical position on the nature of intelligence, being content to define it as the ability to solve new problems, which he recognized as the product of endowment + growth + opportunity. He admitted, too, that intelligence is complex, that there might be different intelligences for dealing with different kinds of problems, though he did not commit himself as to which main types should be distinguished. He tended rather to classify aptitudes in terms of the main kinds of jobs for which people might be selected.

I want, then, to ask again what are the most useful psychological dimensions or factors under which the vocational psychologist can conceptualize people, and how do these originate? What can research tell us of the environmental influences that chiefly contribute to individual differences in these abilities? I intend to argue the case for a model, or structure, of ability factors which, even 3 years ago, might have been considered by most American psychometrists as hopelessly old-fashioned. This is the model based on *g*, the general intellectual factor, plus major and minor group factors. Thurstone's scheme of multiple primary abilities is preferred by almost all psychometrists, though apparently it is seldom adopted by counselors or others who use tests for reaching practical decisions. Despite Thurstone's and Guilford's assurance that general intelligence is too vague and heterogeneous a construct to be worth measuring—we should break it down into its components and measure each individual's profile of factors—most practicing psychologists in schools, clinics, and industry happily go on using the familiar group or individual tests of intelligence. The main concessions they make to the factorist are to obtain separate linguistic and quantitative scores in some academic aptitude tests, and separate verbal and performance scores in the Wechsler scales. When I visited some military psychological establishments in 1957, I was told more than once that military psychologists could not ignore *g*. Try as they would to find differential tests for different army trades, intercorrelations were always so high that recruits appeared to be differentiated more by all-round level of ability than by type of ability, that is to say, by *g* rather than by factor profile. Table 1 provides another instance, extracted from the Psychological Corporation's follow-up studies of the Differential Aptitude Tests. True, these are not pure factor tests, but their aim is to give differential predictions for different educational courses or jobs. I have underlined the four highest validity coefficients in each column, and you will see that the pattern of coefficients for different school courses is sickeningly similar. Verbal and Reasoning tests, that is those which are most typical of the conventional general intelligence test, together with the Numerical test, tend

Table 1. Differential Aptitude Tests: Median Correlations With School Grades Among Several Classes of Ninth-Twelfth-Grade Boys.

| | English | Maths | Science | Social studies |
|---|---|---|---|---|
| Verbal reasoning | .49 | .33 | .54 | .48 |
| Numerical computation | .48 | .47 | .52 | .46 |
| Abstract reasoning | .32 | .32 | .42 | .32 |
| Space | .26 | .26 | .34 | .24 |
| Mechanical comprehension | .21 | .19 | .40 | .21 |
| Clerical speed and accuracy | .22 | .16 | .24 | .21 |
| Spelling | .44 | .28 | .36 | .36 |
| Sentences (English usage) | .50 | .32 | .45 | .43 |

Note. Four highest coefficients in each column are underlined.

to give the best correlations throughout, and only to a limited extent do Space and Mechanical tests add something to the prediction of ability in science courses.

Currently there seems to be greater recognition of the failure of multiple-factor profiles to fulfill their promise, and scepticism over the proliferation of factors. In 1962 Lloyd Humphreys came out in favor of something very similar to the British $g$ + group-factor model, and last year Quinn McNemar (1964) trenchantly criticized the American multiple factorist's "fragmentation of ability, into more and more factors of less and less importance . . . [p. 872]." A general intelligence factor seems unavoidable since substantial positive intercorrelations are found when any cognitive tests are applied to a fairly representative population. But at the same time intelligence has many aspects which can usefully be represented, as Thurstone did, in terms of partially distinct though overlapping primary factors. The trouble arises because any one of these major primaries can be endlessly fractionated, depending simply on the number and variety of different tests in that area which the psychometrist can think up and, I would add, on the homogeneity—the restriction in the range of g—in the tested population. I would entirely agree with Humphreys (1962) that it is useful to superimpose on the hierarchical group-factor model Guttman's notion of facets. Test intercorrelations are affected not only by test content but by the form or technique of the test, its speededness, level of difficulty of the items, whether multiple-choice or creative response, whether analogies, series, or classifications, and so forth. These facets, which are seldom of much diagnostic interest, have been variously referred to as method factors (Campbell & Fiske, 1959), formal factors and work attitudes (Vernon, 1958), instrument factors (Cattell, 1961), and response sets (Cronbach, 1950).

### *Hierarchical Group-Factor Theory*

Figure 1 gives the best indication I can manage of the factors that emerge most consistently when large and varied test batteries are applied to representative samples of adolescents or

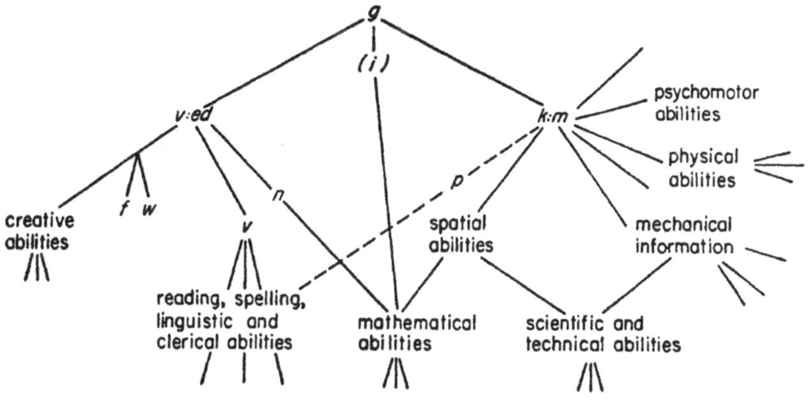


Fig. 1. Diagram of the main general and group factors underlying tests relevant to educational and vocational achievements.

young adults (Vernon, 1961). I admit, of course, that there is no one final structure, since so much depends on the population tested, its heterogeneity and educational background, the particular tests chosen, and the techniques of factorization and rotation employed. I have followed British usage in naming the factors by small letters to differentiate them from the corresponding American primaries from which the *g* element has not been removed.

After removing the general factor (whether by group-factor technique or by rotation of centroid factors), the positive residual correlations always fall into two main groups—the verbal-educational (*v:ed*) group and the spatial-practical-mechanical group. The *v:ed* factor usually yields additional minor fluency and divergent thinking abilities—scholastic and *n* or number subfactors. Likewise the *k:m* complex includes perceptual, physical, and psychomotor, as well as spatial and mechanical factors, which can be further subdivided by more detailed testing. In addition there seem to be various cross-links: For example, clerical tests usually combine verbal ability and perceptual speed, *p;* likewise math and science depend both on number and spatial abilities, *n* and *k*. Sometimes an inductive reasoning ability (also very relevant to science) can be distinguished, though most of the common variance of reasoning tests is apt to be absorbed into *g*. At a still lower level in the hierarchy come what are usually referred to as specific factors, though of course any specific can be turned into an additional narrow group factor by devising additional tests.

Now despite certain differences of analytic technique and interpretation of factors, the hierarchical model and the multiple-factor model are fundamentally in agreement. It is just as legitimate to start, as it were, from the bottom upwards—that is to say, to extract the primaries—and from their intercorrelations calculate the second-order factors, and if need be a third-order factor, corresponding to our major group factors and g. Bernyer (1958) has shown that the two approaches can yield almost identical results. In actual practice, however, rather few multiple-factor analysts (R. B. Cattell, 1963, is a notable exception) bother to allow for obliquity or go on to calculate the higher-order factor loadings of their tests; and when they do so the results are apt to be very inconsistent. British g factor very regularly shows its largest loadings on tests like Progressive Matrices, Shipley Abstraction and Arithmetic Reasoning, whereas American second-order factors appear to have no stable content. Clearly the main reason why you favor multiple factors is that so much of your work is done with rather homogeneous groups like college students or officers in the armed services, where the range of g is so restricted that in effect you only get the group factors which can be rotated to orthogonal simple structure without serious distortion. Several psychometrists, such as Garrett (1946) and Cattell (1963), are inclined to ascribe the lesser prominence of g in these older groups to the differentiation of abilities with age, but there is little doubt that in every piece of research claiming to show such differentiation, the older groups are actually more highly selected, less representative. Take, for example, the recent large-scale survey of Grade 9 to 12 students in Project Talent (Flanagan, Davis, Dailey, Shaycoft, Orr, Goldberg, & Neyman, 1964). I picked out seven of the tests which seemed as different as possible from one another, whose intercorrelations would therefore depend mainly on g, not on common group factors. These were: Farming Information, Memory for Words, English Expression, Creativity, 3-Dimensional Visualization, Arithmetic Computation, and Clerical Checking. At Grade 9 their average intercorrelation among boys was .280, implying that some 28% of their variance could be ascribed to a general factor. By Grade 12 almost every correlation had decreased and the mean was now .241, i.e., some 24% of general variance. However, one notes that the sample at Grade 9 numbered over 39,000, at Grade 12 only 30,000. Clearly more of the duller students would have dropped out by Grade 12, so that the sample was more homogeneous, and this would more than account for the lowered correlations. In the British Army during World War II, with an almost complete spread of ability, correlations between dissimilar tests were if anything higher than those usually found with fourth- to sixth-grade students (Vernon, 1961).

From the point of view of the practical tester, the hierarchical model seems more logical since, in making educational or vocational decisions, he can cover most of the ground just by applying *g* or *g* + *v* tests, and then supplement by spatial-mechanical, clerical, number, or other group-factor tests where relevant. In other words, measures of factors which are higher in the hierarchy generally have better external validity, or more generalizability (Cronbach, Rajaratnam, & Gleser, 1963) to capacities of everyday life; whereas many of the published primary factors seem to be so narrow, so specific to the particular test material, as to have no practical use. This is true, for example, of Thurstone's and other rote memory factors. The user is tempted, even encouraged, to regard them as measuring memorizing ability which is likely to be highly relevant to school learning. In fact they usually correlate with scholastic achievement only insofar as they have not been purified of *g* and *v*. Similarily a large proportion of Guilford's numerous factors of intellect have failed to show any external validity which could not be accounted for by their *g*, *v*, and space content, though I would agree that some of his originality and creativity factor tests may cover a little fresh ground.

Perhaps the basic source of disagreement is that Thurstone and Guilford regarded primary factors almost as fundamental components or chemical elements of the mind, which in combination go to make up all the important human capacities; whereas

Godfrey Thomson (1939), Cyril Burt (1940), and I have always tried to keep in mind that factors are primarily classifications of similar tests. And just because a lot of tests appear to involve memorizing or whatever, and intercorrelate positively, this does not prove that they are good measures of the memorizing that children do in school.

## *Psychological Origins of Factors*

At the same time g theory has its difficulties, in particular that g is not, as Spearman believed, determinate—that is to say, one and the same g whatever cognitive tests one likes to apply. Psychologically it is the all-round level of our thinking skills; while statistically it is merely the average of a battery of tests of intellectual capacities which are so diverse that the group factors or facets involved in each separate test mostly cancel one another out. Hence although we know what kinds of tests are most saturated with g, it can still vary according to the particular measures the psychologist likes to use. Perhaps, though, this is not a serious disadvantage, since it is what one would expect in the light of the psychological contributions of Hebb (1948) and Piaget (1950), Ferguson (1954) and Hunt (1961).

All of these writers point to the need to get away from the notion of intelligence as a definite entity, an autonomous mental faculty, which simply matures as children grow up. Rather we have to think of it in terms of a cumulative formation of more and more complex and flexible schemata (Piaget's term) or phase sequences (Hebb), or what Miller, Galanter, and Pribram (1960) call plans, which develop through interaction between the growing organism and its environment. They depend both upon environmental stimulation and on active exploration and experiment (Piaget's accommodation and assimilation); i.e., they are formed and organized by use. This implies, to a much greater extent than

Piaget seems to have recognized, that they also depend upon personality and motivational factors, organic and social drives, curiosity and interests; and that they are channelled by family, cultural, and educational pressures. Intelligence, then, refers to the totality of concepts and skills, the techniques or plans for coping with problems, which have crystallized out of the child's previous experience. Most representative of these, as Fe guson points out, are the thinking skills which have been overlearned and which are transferable to a wide variety of new situations. Although, of course, each person's accumulation of skills is different, all persons who have been brought up within a fairly homogeneous culture can reasonably be compared at any set of tasks which that culture values and which it likes to include within its conception of intelligence. But obviously, also, the whole structure, from perceptual and linguistic schemata upwards, may differ markedly in other cultures. The group of skills which we refer to as intelligence is a European and American middle-class invention: something which seems to be intimately bound up with puritanical values, with repression of instinctual responses and emphasis on responsibility, initiative, persistence, and efficient workmanship. It is a kind of intelligence which is specially well adapted for scientific analysis, for control and exploitation of the physical world, for large-scale and long-term planning and carrying out of materialistic objectives. It has also led to the growth of complex social institutions such as nations, armies, industrial firms, school systems, and universities, though it has been notably less successful in working out solutions of group rivalries or providing harmonious personal adjustment than have the intelligences of some more primitive cultures. Other cultures have evolved intelligences which are better adapted than ours for coping with problems of agricultural and tribal living. The aboriginal in the Australian desert and the

Eskimo in the Far North have many schemata far more efficient than our own. Again subcultures such as our lower working class, or rural groups, develop rather different intelligence.

How about ability factors other than *g*? It seems entirely plausible that different kinds of skills, or those applied to different kinds of problems, should group together and yield the various group or primary factors that the mental tester discovers. But any reification of such clusters into entities or basic faculties of mind, or what Spearman calls an oligarchic system, is to be deplored. The grouping depends mainly on what cultural and educational pressures dictate. Thus it is very natural, at least in Western cultures, that all the skills bound up with language and school should show a common factor over and above *g*, and that all contrasted skills of a noneducational type should show a different factor. Likewise we can envisage a whole host of minor group factors arising from the overlapping of schemata involved in similar tasks.

### *Cross-Cultural Testing*

Let me now turn to the second half of my title—namely, the environmental influences or other casual agencies that underlie the development of different patterns of abilities. Here, too, the adoption of the hierarchical model simplifies our problem. It would be extraordinarily difficult to inquire into the agencies associated with a large number of Thurstone's primary factors, with Rote Memory, Induction, Fluency, etc., let alone with Guilford's 60 or more factors, since there would be so much overlapping. It seems more feasible to explore the agencies contributing to general intelligence, and those particularly relevant to verbal-educational and to spatial-practical factors—the group factors that carry a lot of everyday-life variance, and to proceed from there to find out what we can about contributory influences to minor factors of, say, creativity, number, art, music, athletic ability, etc., holding intelligence constant.

I would urge that this is a major responsibility of applied psychology in the second half of the twentieth century. If we are to help the newly developing, nontechnological nations of Africa, Asia, South America, and elsewhere, we must know more about the environmental and other handicaps which retard the development of those abilities that are needed for technological advancement (cf. Schwarz, 1961; Vernon, 1962). We want to assist them in selecting children who will make good professionals, teachers, commercial and political leaders, and technicians, and to tell them what factors of diet and health, cultural tradition and family upbringing, and schooling most require attention if they are to produce sufficient highly skilled personnel.

It is in the controversial area of cross-cultural testing that I am at the moment carrying out a series of small-scale researches, supported by the Association for the Aid of Crippled Children. My wife and I have applied a varied battery of tests, mostly individual, to a reference group of 100 11-year-old boys in England, to 50 boys of the same age in Jamaica, and to 90 Canadian Indians and Eskimos; and I hope to sample some African and other cultural groups later. I am confining myself to boys because, as Schaefer and Bayley (1963) point out, the long-term effects of upbringing are more clear-cut than in girls. Also I am working with groups which, by 11 years of age, have acquired enough English to understand oral instructions. Now I am well aware of the difficulties of cross-cultural testing which Anastasi (1958), for example, has discussed; and indeed it follows from what was said earlier that there is no such thing as a culture-free or culture-fair test. But insofar as the developing nations are aiming to achieve viable technological civilizations, they will need Western-type intelligence. Thus it is entirely legitimate to compare their standing with that of Europeans or Americans on tests which are known to sample abilities relevant to Western-type achievements. Moreover, insofar as the contrasted cultures provide a much wider range of environments than commonly occur within Western societies, their test scores should throw a clearer light on the determinants of abilities.

### *Determinants of Test Performance*

Let us broadly distinguish the following classes of determinants:[2]

A. Genetic factors which are nonobservable and nonmeasurable, though we know that they exist since foster children or orphans continue to show some resemblance to their true parents who have had nothing to do with their upbringing. Presumably individuals differ in some quality of the plasticity of the nervous system which makes possible the building up of any schemata or plans; and it may well be that there are genetic differences contributing to linguistic and spatial aptitudes which tend to be sex linked. Certainly there are genetic factors in musical and possibly in mathematical and other talents, however much environment also contributes. One cannot rule out the possibility of genetic differences in aptitudes among ethnic groups or so-called races, but I would agree with the United Nations Educational, Scientific, and Cultural Organization manifesto that we cannot prove them; and they are likely to be small compared with environmentally produced differences.

2. Note the parallel between this classification and Hebb's Intelligence A and B. Elsewhere (Vernon, 1955), I have coined the term "Intelligence C" to refer to actual test results, i.e., to the particular sampling of Intelligence B which an intelligence test provides. Intelligence C also differs from B on account of the facets or instrument factors mentioned above; in other words it is distorted by the C type of determinant.

B. An enormous amount of research, using very varied approaches, has helped to pinpoint the major environmental handicaps to mental development, and I will try to sketch this briefly under nine main headings.

1. Physiological and nutritional factors. These mainly operate during pregnancy and parturition (cf. Stott, 1960); though certain diseases and malnutrition may also be important later insofar as they lower the energy and activity level that the growing child needs to explore his environment and seek out self-stimulating experiences.

2. Perceptual deprivation in the preschool years is suggested by Piaget's and Hebb's work. This may well operate in such situations as Spitz (1945) and Wayne Dennis (1960) describe, but would hardly seem important in most cultural groups where nature provides plenty of sticks, stones, water, and human contacts. I would rather emphasize conceptual deprivation during the school years when parents fail to answer questions, encourage curiosity, and provide books, TV, and other types of experience (cf. Bloom, 1964).

3. Repression of independence and constructive play, either through overprotection, arbitrary subjection, or conformity to tribal traditions. This is very noticeable in West Indian and African societies, and seems to be linked particularly with deficit in spatial abilities, in 3-dimensional perception (cf. Hudson, 1962), and in technical skills. My recent studies with Eskimo boys reveal a strong contrast.

4. Family insecurity and lack of planfulness. In families living at the subsistence level, immediate gratification of hunger and sex needs naturally takes precedence over long-term, purposive planning—the Pleasure Principle over the Reality Principle—and discourages the development of internal controls and rational thinking. In our own culture, Schaefer and Bayley (1963) have

shown the ill effects of parental anxiety, irritability, punitiveness, and rejection on later intellectual as well as social traits.

5. Female dominance. In many cultures, including the West Indian though not the Canadian Indian or Eskimo, the father may take little part in child rearing, and there is a lack of masculine models with whom the boy can identify. According to Witkin's (Witkin, Dyk, Faterson, Goodenough, & Karp, 1962; Witkin, Lewis, Hertzman, Machover, Meissner, & Wapner, 1954) and some other findings, this may favor verbal at the expense of spatial abilities.

6. Education in the underdeveloped countries is often defective, brief or irregular, starved of materials. Teachers may be poorly qualified and they may follow highly formal and mechanical methods, discouraging any intellectual initiative. Yet at the same time even bad education contributes greatly to the development of nonverbal as well as verbal abilities when the average home provides no intellectual stimulation.

7. Linguistic handicaps are almost universal in these societies. There may be a variety of dialects, or a debased and simplified pidgin or Creole; yet English, or sometimes French, is the main medium of instruction, especially for higher education. Unless the child can acquire complete facility in this second language he is likely to be backward in conceptual development and thinking skills, and this too seems to be reflected in nonverbal reasoning as well as in linguistic tests.

8. The conceptual and grammatical structures of the native language may differ markedly from those of English, so that the classifications or relations demanded by a Western-type test may be quite unfamiliar, although the non-Western child can very well classify, relate, and abstract in concrete situations. Again he may never have acquired the ability to interpret pictures as portraying 3-dimensional objects (cf. Biesheuvel, 1952).

9. Adult roles and adolescent aspirations. Here there is little definite evidence. But it is reported of some North American Indian and other cultures that children show fairly normal intellectual development till adolescence, but then, when they realize the depressed status of their minority culture—the absence of opportunity for progress and advancement—apathy sets in. To adapt Gordon Allport's description of personality as "Becoming," intelligence may depend on the future as well as on the past. It is interesting to speculate whether a Western adult does not also cease growing intellectually at 20, 30, 50, or later when he reaches his peak of aspiration and curiosity.

C. This group of determinants obviously overlaps in practice with the B group. But it refers to those characteristics of the test which frequently distort the results of unsophisticated testees, and which could be fairly effectively controlled by appropriate modifications of the form of the test and its administration. Schwarz (1961) has laid down a useful series of principles for getting across Western-type tests to African subjects which, in effect, amounts to teaching them the required mode of response before giving the test. I would still question whether any multiple-choice group test such as Schwarz uses, especially any involving time limits, is suitable for cultures with such different modes of thought and such different attitudes to competition, to working on one's own, or to working at speed.[3] Thus I preferred in my own work to rely more on individual, free-response tests, given like the Terman-Merrill, so that one can expand explanations as necessary and try to ensure that motivation is adequate.

While I hope that this summary of determinants and handi-

3. It is only fair to point out that Schwarz is not concerned with cross-cultural comparisons, but with devising tests which will give useful predictions within African cultures. Thus a speeded test, say, may actually be more predictive of suitability for technical jobs in a culture where speed plays little part in conventional living.

caps provides some clarification, the interpretation of cross-cultural data is still extremely tricky, for test results alone tell us little about what determinants are operating in any particular test. Whiting and Whiting (1960) point out that we may be unaware of the crucial parameters in an unfamiliar culture, and Irvine (1965) argues that different sources of variance may be operating: A particular test may be measuring essentially different things in different cultural contexts. For example, amount and quality of schooling may have very little effect on nonverbal tests like Progressive Matrices, Porteus Mazes, or Draw-a-Man in Western cultures, but may have much greater effects in societies where intellectual stimulation by the home is lacking. However one can hope to make some progress: (*a*) by contrasting a number of different cultures, (*b*) by applying factor analysis within each culture to see how the abilities group and what differences occur in factor patterns, (*c*) by obtaining assessments of major determinants with each culture and observing their correlations with the various test scores or factors.

### *Some Results Obtained in England and the West Indies*

Table 2 indicates the main results of group factor analyses among my English and Jamaican subjects; loadings are shown merely by + or ++ signs, as the detailed figures are available elsewhere (Vernon, 1965). It may be seen that the general pattern is similar in the two groups, though there are some differences in the content of particular tests. In the English group there are a large educational and a subsidiary linguistic factor, a large perceptual-spatial factor, and some separation of the more practical performance tests. With the smaller numbers in the Jamaican sample, these subsidiary factors are less clear-cut, and the only sign of a practical factor is in Porteus Mazes and Formboard. The educational factor is definitely more pervasive,

Table 2. Main Factor Loadings of Tests Given to English and West Indian Eleven-Year Boys.

| Tests | Mean West Indian deviation quotient | English factors | | | | | West Indian factors | | | |
|---|---|---|---|---|---|---|---|---|---|---|
| | | *g* | Educational | Verbal | Perceptual | Practical | *g* | *v:ed* | Perceptual | Practical |
| Arithmetic Achievement | 84 | ++ | + | | | | ++ | + | | |
| Spelling | 94 | + | + | | | | + | + | | |
| Memorizing lists of words | 91 | + | + | | + | | + | + | | |
| English comprehension, usage, spelling | 82 | + | + | + | | | + | + | | |
| Vocabulary, group multiple-choice | 83 | + | + | + | | | + | + | | |
| Vocabulary, individual Terman-Merrill | 72 | + | + | + | | | + | | − | |
| Memorizing oral information | 72 | + | + | | | | + | + | | |
| Abstraction, verbal induction | ?75 | ++ | + | | | | | | | |
| Piaget, arithmetic-orientational | 86 | ++ | | | | | + | + | + | |
| Piaget, visualization-conservation | | + | | | + | + | ++ | | | |
| Matrices, nonverbal induction | 75 | ++ | | | | | ++ | | | |
| Concept formation, sorting test | 90 | + | | + | | | ++ | | | |

| | | | | | | | | |
|---|---|---|---|---|---|---|---|---|
| Porteus Mazes | 91 | + | | | + | + | | + |
| Vernon Formboard | 68 | + | + | + | + | | + | + |
| Kohs Blocks (WISC-Jahoda) | 75 | ++ | + | + | ++ | + | + | |
| Goodenough Draw-a-Man | 91 | + | + | + | + | + | + | |
| Gottschaldt (Embedded) Figures | 88 | + | + | | + | | + | |
| Reproducing Designs (Bender-Gestalt and Terman-Merrill) | 87 | + | + | | + | + | + | |
| Picture Recognition, 3-D Perception | ?85 | + | + | | + | + | | |

Note. + indicates loading of psychological interest, almost all statistically significant; ++ represents loadings of .70 or over. In the second column, certain quotients are preceded by "?" where the identical test was not given to the two groups and an approximate estimate was made.

entering not only into verbal but also most of the paper-and-pencil perceptual tests. Probably it represents general sophistication in understanding instructions and coping with symbolic material, whether verbal or pictorial. The best general factor tests—Piaget, Matrices, and Concept Formation—are those involving the simplest oral instructions and creative responses.

The median Jamaican performance in each test was expressed as a deviation quotient relative to the English distribution, and it will be seen that these figures range from 94 for Spelling down to 68 for Formboard, i.e., from .4 $\sigma$ to 2.1 $\sigma$ below the English mean. Performance is generally best on the more mechanical attainments, though very weak on vocabulary and on information learning, which involve verbal comprehension. The quotients for perceptual tests, including Draw-a-Man, are also mainly around 85–90, and the most serious deficits are in verbal and nonverbal induction, Kohs Blocks, and Formboard—that is in *g* and practical-spatial abilities. This bears out my point that no test can be regarded as culture fair. Jamaican boys actually score better on conventional verbal intelligence and achievement tests, despite their linguistic handicap, than they do on tests which would appear to be purer measures of *g*, or of what Cattell (1963) refers to as fluid ability. I suspect that the same result would be found among Negroes in the United States.

Within each group the environmental variables listed in Table 3 were assessed on the basis of semistructured interviews with the boys and reports from the teachers. Time and expense did not permit home interviews, and in any case I was more interested in home and schooling over the past few years than in the kind of details of early upbringing that Sears, Maccoby, and Levin (1957), Prothro (1961), and others have studied. I would certainly not claim high reliability for these assessments, yet they yielded some quite substantial and plausible correlations with the ability factors. The cultural level of the home is clearly

Table 3. Correlations of Ability Factors with Environmental Variables among English and West Indian Eleven-Year Boys.

| Environmental assessments | English factors | | | | | West Indian factors | | | |
|---|---|---|---|---|---|---|---|---|---|
| | *g* | Educational | Verbal | Perceptual | Practical | *g* | *v:ed* | Perceptual | Practical ? |
| Length and regularity of schooling | −.15 | .31 | | .21 | | .23 | .19 | .26 | |
| Family pattern: unbroken versus broken home | −.11 | .30 | | | .14 | −.17 | .24 | .15 | + |
| Stable home background versus frequent shifts | | | | | | .14 | .17 | | + |
| Economic: parents' job, housing, equipment | .38 | .18 | .24 | | | .27 | .28 | | + |
| Cultural stimulus: books in home, education of relatives, parent interest in education | .56 | .29 | .16 | | | .33 | .46 | .25 | |
| Male dominance and identification versus female overprotection or dominance | | | | | .39 | .25 | | .27 | |
| Initiative and maturity encouraged in play and household activities | .13 | | | .13 | | .27 | .16 | | + |
| Planfulness: rational home climate versus impulsive, emotional, arbitrary | .32 | .26 | | | | .32 | | | |
| Linguistic background | .49 | .31 | .24 | | | .47 | .41 | .28 | |
| Child's health, physical development, and nourishment | | | | | | | .21 | .19 | |

Note. As explained above, no clear practical group factor was established in the West Indian sample. However, Porteus Mazes and Formboard gave substantial positive residual correlations with certain variables, indicated by +.

the most significant single influence—more important than socio-economic rating; and in the Jamaican group, but not the English, it affects perceptual as well as general and educational abilities. Linguistic background is similar, and the planfulness or rationality of the home is particularly associated with *g* factor. Curiously the unbroken home or nuclear family pattern gives slight negative correlations with *g* in both groups, though positive with other factors.[4] Encouragement of initiative, independence, and maturity seems more important in the Jamaican than the English group though it did not relate, as I had hypothesized, to perceptual-practical abilty. But male dominance definitely linked with some aspect of this factor.

During the past 2 months I have been working with groups of boys in Indian reservations in Southern Alberta and Eskimos in the Mackenzie Delta in Arctic Canada. The results are not yet fully scored, let alone analyzed, but they do already bring out one important point—that different groups at similar levels of acculturation, and with similar language difficulties, may show very different patterns of scores. The Eskimos are just about equal to Jamaican standards in written English, though much behind in arithmetic, probably because less stress is laid in Canadian schools on mechanical drill. The Indian boys do somewhat less well on achievement tests; their linguistic handicap is generally greater since less English is spoken in their homes or at school. Like the Jamaicans they are most retarded in oral understanding and vocabulary.

Both groups score much higher than the Jamaicans on Kohs Blocks and other spatial tests, with a mean quotient of 88 instead of 75; and the Eskimos come up very well also on the inductive reasoning tests—Abstraction and Matrices. Now economic con-

4. No explanation can be offered for the slight negative association of schooling with *g* in the English group. In both groups it appears to contribute to spatial as well as to educational development.

ditions are extremely poor in all three groups, and there is similar family instability and insecurity. Thus it seems reasonable to attribute the better performance of Eskimo and Indian groups to the greater emphasis on resourcefulness in the upbringing of boys, perhaps combined with their strong masculine identification. True, the traditional hunting-trapping life is rapidly disappearing and the majority of parents are wage earning or on relief, but the children are still brought up permissively and encouraged to explore and hunt. Moreover, a subgroup of the Eskimos who came from the most isolated Arctic communities scored better on all three of the tests just mentioned than did those who lived in closer contact with whites and had become more acculturated.

Data such as these do not, of course, necessarily prove causality. Thus the correlation between cultural level of the home and intellectual development in the child might arise because brighter parents, who have brighter children, also provide them with better cultural and educational stimulation. Clearly the cross-sectional survey needs to be complemented by longitudinal and, if possible, direct experimental studies. We are on the verge of extremely exciting advances in the understanding and control of intellectual and personality development through such varied approaches as social learning and reinforcement theory, direct observation and follow-up of children, socioanthropological studies, and work such as I have described with mental tests and factor analysis. But I would not claim to have done more than to have scratched the surface, and to have raised many more problems than I have solved.

## *References*

Anastasi, A. *Differential psychology.* New York: Macmillan, 1958.
Bernyer, G. Second order factors and the organization of cognitive functions. *British Journal of Statistical Psychology,* 1958, *11,* 19–29.
Biesheuvel, S. The study of African ability. *African Studies,* 1952, *11,* 45–58, 105–117.
Bingham, W. VanD. *Aptitudes and aptitude testing.* New York: Harper, 1937.
Bingham, W. VanD., & Moore, B. V. *How to interview.* New York: Harper, 1931.
Bloom, B. S. *Stability and change in human characteristics.* New York: Wiley, 1964.
Burt, C. *The factors of the mind.* London: Univer. London Press, 1940.
Campbell, D. T., & Fiske, D. W. Convergent and discriminant validation by the multitrait-multimethod matrix. *Psychological Bulletin,* 1959, *56,* 81–105.
Cattell, R. B. Theory of situational, instrument, second order, and refraction factors in personality structure research. *Psychological Bulletin,* 1961, *58,* 160–174.
Cattell, R. B. Theory of fluid and crystallized intelligence: A critical experiment. *Journal of Educational Psychology,* 1963, *54,* 1–22.
Cronbach, L. J. Further evidence on response sets and test design. *Educational and Psychological Measurement,* 1950, *10,* 3–31.
Cronbach, L. J., Rajaratnam, N., & Gleser, G. C. Theory of generalizability: A liberalization of reliability theory. *British Journal of Statistical Psychology,* 1963, *16,* 137–163.
Dennis, W. Causes of retardation among institutional children: Iran. *Journal of Genetic Psychology,* 1960, *94,* 47–59.
Ferguson, G. A. On learning and human ability. *Canadian Journal of Psychology,* 1954, *8,* 95–112.
Flanagan, J. C., Davis, F. B., Dailey, J. T., Shaycroft, M. F., Ott, D. B., Goldberg, I., & Neyman, C. A. Project TALENT: The American high-school student. Final report, 1964, University of Pittsburgh, Cooperative Research Project No. 635, United States Office of Education.
Garrett, H. E. A developmental theory of intelligence. *American Psychologist,* 1946, *1,* 372–378.
Hebb, D. O. *The organization of behavior.* New York: Wiley, 1948.

Hudson, W. Pictorial perception and educational adaptation in Africa. *Psychologia Africana*, 1962, *9*, 226–239.
Humphreys, L. G. The organization of human abilities. *American Psychologist*, 1962, *17*, 475–483.
Hunt, J. McV. *Intelligence and experience*. New York: Ronald Press, 1961.
Irvine, S. H. Testing abilities and attainments in Africa. *British Journal of Educational Psychology*, 1966, *35*, 24–32.
McNemar, Q. Lost: Our intelligence? Why? *American Psychologist*, 1964, *19*, 871–882.
Miller, G. A., Galanter, E., & Pribram, K. H. *Plans and the structure of behavior*. New York: Holt, 1960.
Piaget, J. *The psychology of intelligence*. London: Routledge & Kegan Paul, 1950.
Prothro, E. T. *Child-rearing in the Lebanon*. Cambridge: Harvard Univer. Press, 1961.
Schaefer, E. S., & Bayley, N. Maternal behavior, child behavior and their intercorrelations from infancy through adolescence. *Monographs of the Society for Research in Child Development*, 1963, *28*, No. 87.
Schwarz, P. A. *Aptitude tests for use in the developing nations*. Pittsburgh, Pa.: American Institute for Research, 1961.
Sears, R. R., Maccoby, E. E., & Levin, H. *Patterns of child rearing*. Evanston, Ill.: Row, Peterson, 1957.
Spitz, R. A. Hospitalism: An inquiry into the genesis of psychiatric conditions in early childhood. *Psychoanalytic Studies of Children*, 1945, *1*, 55–74.
Stott, D. H. Interaction of heredity and environment in regard to "Measured Intelligence." *British Journal of Educational Psychology*, 1960, *30*, 95–102.
Thomson, G. H. *The factorial analysis of human ability*. London: Univer. London Press, 1939.
Vernon, P. E. The assessment of children. In University of London Institute of Education, *Studies in education*. Vol. 7. London: Evans, 1955. Pp. 189–215.
Vernon, P. E. Educational testing and test-form factors. (Res. Bull. 58–3) Princeton, N. J.: Educational Testing Service, 1958.
Vernon, P. E. *The structure of human abilities*. (2nd ed.) London: Methuen, 1961.

Vernon, P. E. Intellectual development in non-technological societies. In G. Nielsen (Ed.), *Proceedings of the XIV International Congress of Applied Psychology*. Vol. 3. *Child and education*. Copenhagen: Munksgaard, 1962. Pp. 94–105.

Vernon, P. E. Environmental handicaps and intellectual development. *British Journal of Educational Psychology*, 1965, 35, pt. 1, pp. 9–20; pt. 2, pp. 117–126.

Whiting, J. W. M., & Whiting, B. B. Anthropological study of child rearing. In P. H. Mussen, *Handbook of research methods in child development*. New York: Wiley, 1960. Ch. 27.

Witkin, H. A., Dyk, R. B., Faterson, H. F., Goodenough, D. R., & Karp, S. A. *Psychological differentiation: Studies of development*. New York: Wiley, 1962.

Witkin, H. A., Lewis, H. B., Hertzmann, M., Machover, K., Meissner, P. B., & Wapner, S. *Personality through perception*. New York: Harper, 1954.

# *Index*

# *Index*

Bei Fragen zur Produktsicherheit wenden Sie sich bitte an:
If you have any questions regarding product safety,
please contact:

Walter de Gruyter GmbH
Genthiner Straße 13
10785 Berlin
productsafety@degruyterbrill.com